THERE ARE ANSWERS TO THE AIDS EPIDEMIC

Acquired Immune D[...] become the most wide[...] [dis]ease of our time. Consider[...] has proved to be resistan[...] [treatments] and therapies. But today, [...] relatively unknown to the general public, there are other ways of combatting this viral infection. *Conquering AIDS Now!* examines the causes of the disease and the recommended methods of prevention. It also provides important information on how to help strengthen the immune system of men and women who have already contracted the AIDS virus.

Conquering AIDS Now! may be the first step on the road to controlling the AIDS virus. It recommends a battery of alternative, all-natural treatments, and offers an inspiring new message of hope, help, understanding, and support.

Scott J. Gregory, N.M.D., Ph.D. is a nutritionist and educator. Raised and educated in Los Angeles, he studied Oriental Medicine at Amherst University in Massachusetts, and at the California Acupuncture College. He also studied biochemistry, nutrition and natural healing in Europe. He is now undertaking advanced research in Oriental Medicine at Emperor College in Santa Monica, California.

Bianca Leonardo, Ph.D. in Nutritional Science (College of Life Science, Austin, Texas), has devoted her life to writing and teaching. She is author of the book *Cancer & Other Diseases Caused by Meat Consumption—Here's the Evidence.* She is Founder and President of the Vegetarian Society, Inc., a non-profit organization dedicated to nutritional education.

CONQUERING AIDS NOW!

With Natural Treatment
A Non-Drug Approach

SCOTT J. GREGORY, N.M.D.
and BIANCA LEONARDO, Ph.D.

Foreword by Alan Cantwell, Jr., M.D.

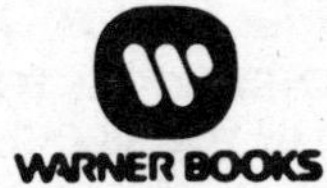

A Warner Communications Company

The material contained in this book is not meant to be a manual for self-treatment, nor should it be a substitute for the advice of a licensed health practitioner. The authors do not diagnose, treat or prescribe, but only educate by using the best information from the best professional sources. In the event you use the information in this book without your health practitioner's approval, you are prescribing for yourself, which is your constitutional right, but the authors and publisher assume no responsibility.

Warner Books Edition

Copyright © 1986 Tree of Life Publications
All rights reserved.

This Warner Books edition is published by arrangement with
Tree of Life Publications, 513 Wilshire Blvd., #244
Santa Monica, CA 90401

Warner Books, Inc., 666 Fifth Avenue, New York, NY 10103
A Warner Communications Company
Printed in the United States of America
First Warner Books Trade Paperback Printing: October 1987
10 9 8 7 6 5 4 3 2 1

Library of Congress Cataloging-in-Publication Data
Gregory, Scott J.
      Conquering AIDS now.

      Reprint. Originally published: Conquering a
modern plague. Santa Monica, CA: Tree of Life
Publications, c1986.
            Bibliography: 5 pp.
            Includes index.
            1. AIDS (Disease)—Treatment.   2. Holistic
medicine.   I. Leonardo, Bianca.   II. Title.
[DNLM: 1. Acquired Immunodeficiency Syndrome—
therapy—popular works.   WD 308 G823c 1986a]
RC607.A26G75   1987   616.97'92   87-10530
ISBN 0-446-38733-9 (pbk.) (U.S.A.)
            0-446-38734-7 (pbk.) (Canada)

ATTENTION: SCHOOLS AND CORPORATIONS

Warner books are available at quantity discounts with bulk purchase for educational, business, or sales promotional use. For information, please write to: Special Sales Department, Warner Books, 666 Fifth Avenue, New York, NY 10103.

ARE THERE WARNER BOOKS YOU WANT
BUT CANNOT FIND IN YOUR LOCAL STORES?

You can get any Warner Books title in print. Simply send title and retail price, plus 50¢ per order and 50¢ per copy to cover mailing and handling costs for each book desired. New York State and California residents, add applicable sales tax. Enclose check or money order—no cash, please—to: Warner Books, PO Box 690, New York, NY 10019. Or send for our complete catalog of Warner Books.

DEDICATION

We dedicate this book to "Sunny," Bianca's son, who lost his life at age ten; to Scott's mother and father, who early left this life (all in hospitals); and to the other millions of human beings everywhere who prematurely—and in pain and suffering—left this world—because of a lack of knowledge of Natural Health and Healing.

May they not have lived—or died—in vain.

We also dedicate this book to Dr. Norman Walker, who died a natural death, in his sleep, on June 6, 1985, at the age of 109. He was a pioneer in the field of Natural Health and Healing. We love him and honor him.

Finally, we dedicate this book to the medical doctors and other health practitioners who see the light and are striving to show humanity the true road to health.

Scott J. Gregory and Bianca Leonardo

ACKNOWLEDGMENTS

We wish to thank the following for their contributions to this book:

Anna Thea Bogdanovich, photographer, who painstakingly took the pictures for the photo section; Eric Small and the other models; Alan J. Cantwell, Jr., M.D., for the foreword; and Robert S. Mendelsohn, M.D., who appreciates our work.

We thank many health practitioners and authors for the knowledge we have gained over the years from them, and thank God (sometimes called the Universal or Divine Mind), for the ideas sent to us for this book. We are only channels for the inspiration that comes from the divine consciousness; so are all men and women who do anything creative or noble, whether they know it or not.

May our work bless all who come into contact with it.

CONTENTS

CONTENTS — PHOTO SECTION

Causes of Disease

Symptoms of Disease

Natural Treatment

FOREWORD

by Alan Cantwell, Jr., M.D.

AIDS (Acquired Immune Deficiency Syndrome) is the most serious epidemic disease of our time. A recent poll indicated that the number one fear of most Americans is contracting cancer. AIDS is second.

Five years ago, most people had never heard of the disease, and only a few doctors had ever seen a case. In 1981, when the epidemic officially began in America, AIDS was thought to be solely a disease of homosexuals (''the gay plague''). By 1982, drug addicts, hemophiliacs, and Haitians were also found to be at high risk for AIDS. Later, infants of drug-addicted and promiscuous mothers, and people who received infected blood transfusions were added to the list. By 1985, a media blitz surrounding Rock Hudson's death from AIDS brought world-wide attention to the disease.

In 1984, a new virus was discovered in the blood of

most, but not all, AIDS patients. This new, sexually transmitted AIDS virus is called the HIV virus (Human Immunodeficient Virus) and is considered by most scientists to be the sole cause of AIDS. The HIV virus can seriously damage the immune system by selectively killing off "T-cells." These white blood cells of the immune system are vital in the body's defense against infectious microbes. When the discovery of the new AIDS virus was announced in April 1984, it was predicted that a protective vaccine would be developed against the virus within two years. However, it was quickly discovered that the virus mutated, making a vaccine impossible before 1990, at the earliest.

"No effective vaccine is commercially available for *any* germ of the retrovirus family" (including the AIDS virus), state James I. Slaff, M.D., and John K. Brubaker, in the book *The AIDS Epidemic,* published by Warner Books, Inc., in 1985.

There are two major diseases which are characteristic of AIDS: Kaposi's sarcoma and *Pneumocystis carinii* pneumonia. Kaposi's sarcoma is a form of cancer first recognized over a century ago in Europe. For many decades, Kaposi's sarcoma has been a very common form of cancer in children and heterosexual adults in Central Africa. A very high percentage of Central Africans have already been infected by the HIV virus.

Pneumocystis carinii pneumonia is caused by a parasite. This "opportunistic" lung disease has been known for over a half century. Previous epidemics of Pneumocystis pneumonia in newborns and infants were prevalent in Central Europe during the 1940s and 1950s. Originally the disease was believed to be caused by a virus. Two decades later, pathologists finally learned how to see the parasite in diseased tissue by using a proper stain for their microscopic examinations. Mini-epidemics of Pneumocystis pneumonia were recorded in cancer wards in America during the 1960s and 1970s, particularly in children treated for cancer with chemotherapy. The Pneumocystis parasite primarily attacks people with weakened immune systems. Pneumocystis pneumonia is the most frequent cause of death in AIDS patients.

As of September 1986, we are told that about 1,000 persons per day are getting this disease, nationally. It is estimated that many more get ARC (AIDS-related complex). Two babies per day are born with AIDS in New York City.

The fear of AIDS which now pervades society has drastically changed the sexual and social behavior of millions of Americans, both ''gay'' and ''straight.'' AIDS experts advise that all sexually active people should practice ''safe sex'' unless they have been in a monogamous relationship for at least five years. It is widely believed that sex with a person who is carrying the AIDS virus can literally be ''the kiss of death.''

What can we do to protect ourselves? Obviously, more care must be taken in the sexual areas of life. Greater attention to personal hygiene is mandatory for sexual partners. Sexual promiscuity is now fraught with danger as never before. Unprotected anal intercourse appears to be the most risky form of sexual activity. Drug abuse has been closely linked to AIDS in the majority of cases. Cocaine, ''recreational'' and ''designer'' drugs used as sexual stimulants, as well as the inhalation of ''poppers'' (butyl nitrite), are clearly damaging to the immune system.

There is growing evidence to suggest that the new AIDS virus attacks people whose immune systems are already weakened. For this reason, concerned individuals should make every effort to eat properly and pay attention to nutrition, avoid stress as much as possible, get adequate rest, limit the number of sexual partners, and avoid excesses of drugs, tobacco, and alcohol.

Although most AIDS experts believe that the new HIV virus is the cause of AIDS, there are some physicians, like myself, who believe that AIDS is simply another form of infectious cancer brought about in most instances by a sexually promiscuous or a drug-oriented lifestyle, or both. This view is supported by a recent autopsy study of 52 patients who died from AIDS, which proved that the Kaposi's sarcoma form of cancer could be detected in over 94% of these patients, although apparently only one-third of the AIDS patients develop cancer. My belief is that AIDS and cancer are both caused by infectious cancer bacteria.

There are important reasons why scientists downplay the clear association between AIDS and cancer. The most obvious reason is that AIDS has shattered the myth that cancer is never contagious or transmissible through sexual contact. The Public Health Service has recommended since 1983 that sexual contact be avoided with persons showing evidence of Kaposi's sarcoma, the common cancer in AIDS.

It is now painfully apparent that orthodox medicine has no satisfactory treatment for AIDS. There is no available drug that eliminates the AIDS virus from infected individuals, nor are there drugs which repair the damaged immune system in AIDS. Anti-cancer chemotherapy has been a dismal failure for Kaposi's sarcoma. Chemotherapy further depresses the immune system and increases the risk of life-threatening infections in AIDS patients. Similarly, the standard drug treatment of opportunistic infections in AIDS patients often fails because drugs simply do not work when the immune system is weak.

So what do we do? As we have done for cancer, we must now strive for PREVENTION of AIDS. For those unfortunate people with a life-threatening diagnosis of AIDS or AIDS-related disease, it is mandatory that any unhealthy lifestyle habits be exchanged for a lifestyle that emphasizes healthy living and positive thinking.

Persons with AIDS must bear the burden of assuming the major responsibility for their healing.

We have all lived in the modern age of medicine. We get sick—we go to the doctor, expecting him to heal us. With AIDS, it is no longer that kind of ballgame. With AIDS, we must develop new methods of treatment, and develop a greater understanding of AIDS if we are to heal persons with this dread disease. Many people who have awaited the latest miracle drug for AIDS are now dead and buried.

My own scientific views of the orthodox medical treatment of AIDS have been shattered by watching friends die of AIDS. Death from AIDS is too horrible to describe, and there is no point in concentrating on death. We must focus on life and wellness and new ways of living and loving in the age of AIDS.

Many years ago, Edgar Cayce, the famous psychic and healer, said: ''What we eat and what we think make what we are, both physically and mentally.'' I believe there is much truth in Cayce's holistic views on keeping the body healthy by proper diet, nutrition, and above all, proper mental attitude with the ''Mind as the Builder.''

In this book, there are many ideas on strengthening the immune system and healing the body, particularly through nutrition and other natural therapies. Undoubtedly, some of these ideas might be considered heretical to some readers, or as magical, mystical, and metaphysical to others. People with AIDS are desperately in need of miracles. We hope to supply them with a few sparks of collective wisdom to further them along their journey to wellness.

Although physicians play the traditional role of healers in our culture, we should never forget that we are all healers. We have the capacity to heal ourselves and to heal others. We must also allow ourselves to accept healing from others. We must never forget that all of us, without exception, are worthy of being healed. At a deeper level, we are all aware of the Source of all healing.

Everyone who has ideas about AIDS should be heard. There is much to learn about this disease. No doubt, the epidemic will affect our sexual lives for many years to come, and will also teach us much about our capacity to love one another during this AIDS crisis.

This book contains messages of help, hope, support, and understanding to those who are ill with AIDS and other life-threatening diseases. Most importantly, I sense the authors have an underlying message of love.

Although it may sound trite, I am convinced that love is the best medicine we currently have for AIDS. Unfortunately, I cannot give a scientific definition of love because I am still trying to understand what love is. As a physician and scientist, I like to consider love as something which seems to help people who give it freely and those who accept it with joy.

Alan Cantwell, Jr., M.D.
Los Angeles, California
September, 1986

"C.A.N." UPDATE—A NEWSLETTER

"C.A.N." stands for "CONQUERING AIDS NOW!"—and is the title of a new monthly newsletter. It is dedicated to positive news on the subject.

Nutritional and other vital health information of interest to *anyone*, and the latest news on AIDS is covered.

The emphasis is the same as that of this book —alternative, natural therapies and prevention.

It has been said that AIDS has the potential of ending America as we know it by the next century. This makes AIDS one of the most important diseases of our age. The big questions are: Is AIDS polluting humanity's bloodstream? Could it eventually decimate humanity?

The reader is invited to subscribe and help to: CONQUER AIDS NOW!

For further information, write:

TREE OF LIFE
P. O. Box 5688
Santa Monica, CA 90405

DRUGS USED IN THE TREATMENT OF AIDS

(1) Trimethoprim
(2) Sulfamethoxazole
(3) Pentamidine isethionate
(4) Ribavirin (a flu drug used in 70 or more countries)
(5) Suramin (a long-popular drug used to treat parasitic diseases like African sleeping sickness)
(6) Trisodium phosphonoformate (a Swedish drug used for herpes)
(7) Azidothymidine (AZT)—a new, unusually potent anti-viral drug
(8) HPA-23 (the mineral compound used in Paris to treat actor Rock Hudson)

None of these drugs cures AIDS, and all are fairly toxic and produce debilitating side effects, such as kidney and liver damage.

Many drugs are being tested on humans—e.g., Alpha-interferon, interleukin-2, and IMREG-1.

NATURAL, LIFE-SAVING HEALTH PRACTICES

1. Natural Foods
2. Food Combining for Maximum Absorption
3. Natural Supplementation Therapy
4. Catalytic Vitamins
5. Herbal Therapies
6. Lymphatic Cleansing
7. Intestinal Cleaning and Implantation
8. Hydrotherapy
9. The Sauna
10. Fever, Artificially Induced
11. Massage (turns on adrenal function)
12. Dry Brush Massage
13. Stress Reduction
14. Acupuncture
15. Exercise
16. Fresh Air
17. Adequate Rest and Sleep
18. Sunlight Therapy
19. Creative Visualization
20. Meditation and Prayer

ONE

SUCCESS WITH AIDS

This is a book about AIDS. But it is not just about the disease, or even about homosexuality. It is about re-education and regeneration.

Through education, the reader can learn a more natural, healthful way of living. We, the authors, also hope to inspire AIDS patients to cope with the fear the disease is generating. A body cannot heal itself or be healed by anything if the mind is totally taken over by fear.

AIDS is a disease brought about by modern social and environmental factors. Our modern culture tempts mankind toward a continuous trip in the "fast lane." It also enthralls us with a poor quality of air, food, and water, and chemicals of all kinds. How can we help but be weakened by all of these pollutants in our environment? And AIDS is found mostly in large cities, centers of such pollution.

AIDS strikes people who are admitted homosexuals with

more frequency. Many homosexuals live with far more stress in their lives than heterosexuals. AIDS sufferers probably use more illegal drugs than other persons. (See pages 32–34 in this book.)

All of us are taught by the media to use specific chemical remedies to cure specific ailments. These drugs do mask the ailments (for a while). And fast foods, with artificial ingredients, do stop our hunger (but aren't nutritious). However, these are *not* the solutions to peoples' health problems.

Chemotherapy and radiation are the orthodox treatments for both cancer and AIDS. But these treatments wipe out dangerous cells without regard for healthy neighboring cells. Antibiotics may be a co-factor in the development of AIDS, says Dana Ullman, homeopathic doctor and researcher. (See Chapter 9, "Other Viewpoints.")

The natural, alternative methods and therapies suggested in this book help neutralize the factors that make modern lifestyles the "high risk" avenues for AIDS to appear.

But the natural therapies presented here do exact a price. As the universe is based on balance, one will need to balance his getting well by giving up some aspects of his current lifestyle. He will have to make some changes. Will it be worth it? We think so.

Any extreme changes in the therapeutic modalities (allopathic intervention—chemotherapy, radiation, antibiotics, etc.) may hinder healing. Changes must be gradual, but the problem is—with AIDS patients—there is not much time.

In 1983–84, a number of men came to me (Scott Gregory) who had been diagnosed by M.D.s as having the Acquired Immune Deficiency Syndrome. The medical doctors told some of them that their chances of recovery were very slim, and there was no hope; there was nothing they could do but die. I shared with them the natural methods now presented in this book. I did not diagnose, treat, or prescribe, but only educated them to help improve their general health. After the men had decided that they wanted to change their health habits, and acted on the recommendations, their health did improve. In fact, upon returning to their doctors, they were pronounced "clear" or in remission.

Mr. A., a bisexual actor in his late 20's, came to see me with his girlfriend. He had many symptoms, and was frantic and desperate. He described to me these symptoms: nausea, diarrhea, sore throat, loss of appetite, an altered sense of taste, lactose intolerance and intolerance to foods that he had been eating regularly, a bad taste in the mouth, belching, digestive upsets, a feeling of fullness after eating very little, weight loss, a dryness of the oral and mucous membranes and tongue, a soreness of the mouth and tongue and burning feeling in the mouth, night sweats, extreme fatigue, dehydration, physical weakness, headaches, depression, a general rundown feeling and blurred vision.

Observable symptoms were: furry, white coating on the tongue, blood in the stool, persistent shortness of breath accompanied by a persistent, dry cough. (Pulmonary problems are commonly seen in AIDS patients.) Other visible symptoms were: he was easily bruised (caused by a decreased number of platelets—cells essential to the clotting of the blood), swollen lymph nodes, especially in the groin, neck, and underarm areas.

Other symptoms AIDS patients show are: infections due to *Pneumocystis carinii*, cytomegalovirus, Candida Albicans (yeast infection), herpes, and toxoplasma. Also: neurological problems, enlarged and discolored nodules, plaques on the skin, and Kaposi's (purple) sarcoma on the skin.

Mr. A. had all the symptoms except the sarcoma. Although I was not familiar with AIDS at the time, I suggested a change of lifestyle, an improved nutrition, cleansing herbs, supplements, and a lymphatic cleaning— to improve his general health. (See Chapter 5—"Natural Treatment, The Gregory Method"—of this book.)

Mr. B., in his early 40's, was not as sick as Mr. A. His manner, dress and style of speaking were very casual. His symptoms were not so extreme, and he was rather matter-of-fact in his questions. He had been sent by a holistic doctor, an acupuncturist. He had a history of many infections, including Type-A hepatitis. His major complaints were: swollen lymph nodes (which seem to be visible with any systemic infection), digestive upset, lack of appetite, sinusitis (stuffed nose), and difficulty with breathing. He also had been diagnosed by a medical doctor as having AIDS.

Mr. B. used some of these natural methods and improved markedly. It took eight weeks for him to recover. He had a blood test; the AIDS was declared "in remission." He stopped drinking alcohol and embarked upon a healthful lifestyle. When I saw him two years later, he was still well.

Mr. C. was a cocaine user and a braggart concerning his sexual prowess, with both men and women. His symptoms were: painful urination, discharges, diarrhea and constant fatigue. He was extremely aggressive and hyperactive. His condition worsened and he was in great pain. Then he became amenable to the natural program. The course of the disease was less difficult and less painful than in other cases, and he got good results. It took him longer to get "clear"—about ten weeks.

Mr. D. was a young dancer, a professional with a great future. Upon learning that he had AIDS, he decided to go to a conventional hospital as an outpatient, during which time chemotherapy and radiation were used. Side effects resulted—hair loss, radiation poisoning, a jaundiced skin, a total lack of vitality, organ problems, etc. (All drugs seem to destroy liver cells, and they kill good cells as well as bad cells.)

At that point he decided to try natural methods. The lymphatic system was cleansed, ridding the body of pathogens, and the toxic chemicals and drugs that were complicating the problem. With the natural program, the body can start to heal itself and become healthy, as Nature intended.

Mr. E. was a businessman, well-dressed, very sophisticated, in his early 30's. Superficially, he showed no symptoms of AIDS and looked well, but had severe rectal bleeding. I asked him if he had hemorrhoids or some type of rectal irritation. He had much blockage in his stomach, and had problems with digestion and absorption. I advised him to see a physician, who pronounced that he had AIDS.

After a time, he returned to me, and decided to "go natural." Recovery was very speedy. In time, his physician pronounced him "clear"—as with the other cases.

Each time I saw him, he was smiling and happy. He knew he would overcome the disease, and did—indicating the power of the mind in healing and recovery.

This type of individual can spread the disease, but does not get a full-blown case of the symptoms himself. This is called a sub-clinical case.

There have been other cases of success with AIDS across the nation, but I am describing only five cases here, from my own experience.

All the individuals I treated were in a depleted and sickened state, with a low resistance, susceptible to infections. Some of them had other "opportunistic infections" before AIDS. These are caused by organisms commonly found in the environment which the healthy immune system resists, so we are told. When the immune system is not functioning properly, these organisms seize the "opportunity" to infect the body.

The true causes of disease have been known for years, in the natural health movement. They are to be found in our denatured environment and health-destroying mode of living; carcinogenic (cancer-producing) substances in our air, soil, water and food; drug addiction; overindulgences of all kinds: excessive protein, and the body's inability to properly utilize it; nutritional deficiencies and other physical and emotional stresses which weaken and break down the body's resistance to diseases, a genetic predisposition, etc.

It is also evident that the battle against AIDS can be won only by massive preventive programs aimed at eliminating all environmental carcinogenic factors, improving our nutritional patterns, which strengthen our immune functions, consequently strengthening the body's resistance to disease.

When AIDS is already manifested, the only program of treatment that will lead to success must be all-encompassing and supportive so that the body can heal itself.

The supportive measures, as described in this book, include lymphatic and internal cleansing, artificially induced fever, a carcinogen-free diet, nutritional support, herbal and vitamin supplementation—all aimed at inhibiting the development of AIDS and helping the body to heal itself.

Are Waerland, a Swiss doctor, said: "We do not deal with disease—only with mistakes in our way of living."

TWO

THE CAUSES OF DISEASE

The new frontiers of enlightened thought are discovering that diseases are of man's own making. They are the end result of a longtime abuse in the form of poor living habits, faulty nutrition, and other health-destroying environmental factors.

Man's disregard of these laws in respect to his environment, nutrition, and physical and emotional needs leads to disharmony—disease.

Natural healing is not a new philosophy or passing fad. It is at least as ancient as that great doctor of antiquity, Hippocrates, in Greece (B.C.)—who is called "the father of medicine," but whose principles are followed little today by the medical profession.

Natural healing was rediscovered in our time by a number of great thinkers and pioneers in the field of health. It is a true science based on the principle of intelligent support of the natural healing power inherent in the living organism.

Lasting results can be attained only when a wise doctor (or a patient with wisdom) assists and supports the body's own healing forces, which institute the health-restoring processes and accomplish the actual cure. Natural therapies are directed at correcting the underlying causes of the disease, strengthening the patient's resistance and creating the most favorable conditions for the body's own healing to take place.

Man's body is endowed with an enormous capacity to adapt itself to abnormal, adverse conditions. But this capacity is limited. When health-destroying conditions continue unchecked for prolonged periods of time, various disturbances in the functions of the organs and glands begin to manifest themselves. These may be in the form of fever, repeated colds and infections, tonsilitis, an enlarged liver, increased blood pressure, skin eruptions, etc. In most instances, these are protective and defensive measures initiated by the organism in its effort to protect itself against the existing abnormal conditions. Suppressed by drugs, such symptoms may get progressively worse or change their nature and ultimately result in chronic pathological and degenerative changes. This may be how AIDS develops.

It is becoming increasingly evident that the present-day medical approach, with drugs treating isolated symptoms, is unable to solve the problem of the catastrophic increase in the degenerative diseases—above all, AIDS and also cancer, cardiovascular disorders, arthritis, diabetes, etc. The conventional approach of treating symptoms with specific drugs or other material remedies, without taking into consideration the patient's total condition of health and correcting the underlying causes of his ill health, is as unscientific as it is ineffective. A more fundamental approach takes man's environmental factors, nutritional patterns, and mental and emotional attitudes into consideration.

Treatment in natural healing is directed toward the elimination of the basic cause of disease. It helps the body's own healing activity and restores the equilibrium and harmony in the function of the vital organs.

Our philosophy is based on the fundamental principle of intelligent cooperation with nature. Natural healing sees man as a part of nature, subject to its eternal laws. It incorporates all the harmless and effective therapies that can be applied in the correction of ill health. Diseases can be cured only by the body's own inherent healing power.

AIDS patients can be helped when a therapist or the patient himself assists these healing forces, and creates the most favorable conditions for the healing processes to succeed.

Where surgery is needed because of accidents or other causes, it should be used. Where there is damage or dislocation in the spine or the joints, chiropractic treatments should be applied.

Where the disease is caused by SYSTEMIC DISORDERS and BIOCHEMICAL IMBALANCES due to faulty eating and living habits—the corrective nutritional and naturopathic healing methods should be used.

Spiritual healing and the psychological approach are also valuable. The power of spiritual and psychological therapies has been explored only slightly. The power of the mind is a vast, unexplored territory—and is the next great frontier to conquer in healing. It was used in Biblical times and by primitive tribes (who called on the Great Spirit, and also used herbs and other elements of nature). But the civilized world gives all power to matter (as in drugs) for the most part. It largely ignores the power of Mind — but the time will come when this will change — and mankind will be greatly benefitted.

Within the field of biological medicine, there are collective and natural explanations for the causes of illness. There are many causes, intimately interrelated. Heredity and environment are common ones.

Heredity can lead to the development of certain diseases, either directly, as in the case of hemophilia, or by providing predisposition, in which case a number of other factors must also be present before a disease will appear.

Environmental factors include such things as bacteria, the working place, physical causes such as radiation and accidents, and the psychological — e.g., dislike of one's work.

This approach to disease lends another dimension to the question of health and disease, where the responsibility for one's health falls primarily on the individual. We must take care of our bodies, eat a healthful diet, improve our emotional and mental attitudes, and follow other natural laws of health.

Here are some co-factors that cause disease, or lower resistance to disease. Many of them are within our power to change:

Co-Factors Causing Disease

1. Malnutrition: insufficient and/or devitalized foods. A poor diet overloads the body with toxins. They, in turn, must be neutralized by the immune system, which causes it to become overworked. We recommend a natural diet and a food plan that is rotated and progressive. (As the body gains health, new foods are added.)

2. Mechanical, physical and chemical irritations: anal intercourse, the use of drugs, tobacco, alcohol, etc.

3. Diethylstilbestrol is a major causative factor. "DES" is an artificial female sex hormone, widely used in meat production—for more profit (it causes the animals to fatten faster, and the cows to constantly lactate, to produce huge quantities of milk).

It is estimated that 85% of all meat in the U.S. contains dangerous residues of Diethylstilbestrol.

"DES" feminizes men: it destroys both fertility and the sexual libido in men.

Author Scott Gregory was brought up on a heavy meat diet. Eating meat three times a day was customary. Being sensitive, he became hyperactive because of the heavy meat consumption. (The body must expel the uric acid and ammonia by-products of human metabolism. Activity helps excrete these poisons.) Scott would get extremely aggressive, especially after eating chicken. As he matured, he found that the excessive consumption of animal protein overstimulated the hormonal secretions, and hence, sexual desires.

In interviewing Persons With AIDS, the authors found *other* men who had the same experience. One man told the authors that his father was a butcher, the family ate meat three times a day, and from an early age he was overstimulated sexually.

The macrobiotic philosophy holds the same concept—that meat overstimulates. Excessive eating of meat and other cholesterol-rich foods not only contributes to arteriosclerosis, but impairs blood circulation and diminishes the oxidation of cells, increasing the risk of AIDS.

4. Artificial sweeteners—cyclamates and saccharins (found in diet soft drinks, e.g.). These cause digestive disorders, which result in auto-immune deficiency, climaxing in AIDS.

5. Smog—impure air. Ozone, carbon monoxide, nitrogen dioxide and other photo-chemical pollutants in smog, that now cover the cities of this country. Chemicals present in smog cause many health disorders. These are physical irritants. Smog makes our eyes burn and water; you can imagine what it does to our lungs and the rest of our bodies.

6. Coal tar dyes, highly toxic, are used in foods, soft drinks, cosmetics, and medicine.

7. Radioactive chemicals. Radiation is all around us. Strontium 90 has been found in cow's milk. From atomic testing, this harmful substance gets into the food chain. Cows eat the contaminated grass, and we drink their milk.

Iodine 131 is another radioactive chemical. It is particularly dangerous to people who consume large quantities of milk—especially children.

8. Excessive X-rays. X-rays are overused these days; overuse is harmful.

9. Cadmium is toxic in large amounts. It reaches us from automobile exhaust fumes, fertilizers, and industrial wastes. It pollutes the soil and the water and is taken up by plants—particularly cereal grains.

10. Rancid foods and oils. Whole foods maintain their integrity. Modern food processing and marketing methods, resulting in "long shelf life," produce foods that are stale and rancid. We must also watch some of the natural, unprocessed, so-called health foods. Fractionated foods, such as wheat flour, nut butter and wheat germ oil, are often rancid. Natural, unprocessed foods are extremely perishable. Wheat germ, for example, will turn rancid in a couple of days. Rancid foods are extremely dangerous; not only are they deficient in vitamins, such as A, E, and F, but during the process of becoming rancid, extremely harmful substances, such as peroxides, are formed. Being strong chemical irritants, they can cause sickness.

11. Concurrent infections; other underlying related diseases.

12. Genetic variations and weaknesses.

13. Poor health habits and uncleanliness.

14. Exhaustion; depression; anxiety; insufficient rest and sleep; stress.

15. Overexposure to the sun's rays.

16. Foreign antigens (substances that are foreign to the body, that stimulate the production of antibodies). Some are: proteins, bacteria, pollen, etc. The immune system is becoming weakened and overworked.

Toxemia, Disease and Health

Cells require oxygen. When the body gets clogged up with toxic accumulations, cell respiration becomes impeded. Over-eating, over-drinking, poor food combining (see food combining section in this book), create putrified wastes that must be expelled. Generally, a normal, healthy body can detoxify these wastes. It is when we become gluttonous, and eat devitalized food, that our digestive system becomes over-stressed. If food is quickly and efficiently absorbed, the body can use the resulting energy to rebuild body tone, rid itself of stored toxins, and to heal itself. Health authorities in the medical and biochemical fields now recognize that all the foreign substances we take in daily, including synthetic, processed and contaminated foods, are the causes of many degenerative diseases.

A healthful diet consists of at least 60% high-moisture-content foods, mostly fruits and vegetables. These cause the expelling of toxic, metabolic wastes from the system. Much of our sickness is brought upon us by germs that feed on these wastes. The presence of a germ in the body does not indicate that it is the cause of sickness, because germs are present in a healthy body.

When our bodies cannot take any more toxins, they rebel with fever, diarrhea, sweating, swollen lymph nodes, etc. We are told that fever is dangerous and we are immediately given more toxins, namely, drugs. This stops the natural detoxification process. Yes, people do die of high fever and diarrhea; nevertheless, the body has a tremendous healing potential of its own, which for the most part is not trusted; therefore, the natural healing is not allowed to occur.

All of our orifices have specialized filters, both mechanical and chemical. When we are healthy, they protect us from foreign invasions. In short, all the toxins we consume and allow to enter our bloodstream, what we allow to be done to us—fear, worry and other negative emotions—all these cause disease.

What must we do to get well?

(1) Resolve the toxic substances within. The techniques are given throughout this book.

(2) Reframe thought patterns and negative emotions. (See ''Other Viewpoints'': Anthony Robbins's technique.)

(3) Learn about nutrition—the truth about foods—harmful or wholesome. Read labels on containers. Educate yourself and find out what is best for you. To give blanket recommendations is not correct counselling. We are all individuals, with individual and special needs.

Author Scott J. Gregory has been on his deathbed twice, and totally recovered, in spite of medical intervention. Amidst great trials, he learned this lesson:

WE HAVE TO TAKE RESPONSIBILITY FOR OUR OWN SICKNESS. And—THE PATIENT MUST BE ALLOWED TO DECIDE ON THE MODE OF TREATMENT HE DESIRES; it is against freedom of conscience to be forced to take treatments in hospitals that one does not believe in, or approve of, and that one believes will harm oneself.

THREE

THE CAUSES OF AIDS

Why are people getting AIDS today? Why did we not hear of it in the past? There are at least two reasons:

The germ or pathogen has become resistant, due to medical intervention. It is a super-strong microbe. By "medical intervention" we are referring to the chemicals being given, especially antibiotics. They create a more aggressive, virulent pathogen which appears to be indestructible.

AIDS is a lifestyle disease, the result of an abuse of the body. This is not a moral judgment, but a fact.

When being "gay" became more acceptable and new "recreational" drugs became easily obtained, the social mores changed, and so did the sexual practices—dramatically. Chemical sex "enhancers" (amyl nitrite and "poppers"); hard drugs plus a heavy use of alcohol and late hours—all these take their toll on health.

Amyl nitrite was originally used in medicine as a heart stimulant. It is now used for a sexual high. There are many synthetic drugs made in illegal laboratories that are being sold and sniffed, injected, or consumed—all making for a destructive lifestyle.

AIDS is not so prevalent among older gays. As we get older, our immune function weakens. So why are the older men not getting AIDS? Possibly because they cannot keep up with the fast pace of the younger men.

AIDS is not only one disease; it is an infection which develops into immune suppression, which results in a cancer.

Many AIDS victims had previously been infected with Hepatitis B and other diseases which activated and weakened immune response, with a long history of infection.

Nor does AIDS have only one cause. Sexual promiscuity and over-activity, drug abuse and alcohol, and combinations of these that compound the harmful effects—all are causes.

"Now no one is safe from AIDS"—headline on the cover of a national weekly. THIS IS NOT TRUE.

"Only 10% of the people that are exposed to the virus develop symptoms of AIDS," states Dr. J. A. Levine of the University of California, San Francisco.

Then what causes the 10% to develop the symptoms of AIDS?

Most scientific information today suggests that AIDS (Acquired Immune Deficiency Syndrome) is caused by the weakening of the immune system.

The immune system is the defense team of your body. When intact, it protects you twenty-four hours a day —against chemicals in the environment, drugs and other foreign substances entering the body, and your own body cells—if they have been transformed into malignant cells. The defect in the immune system caused by the AIDS infection results in the improper function of T-lymphocyte cells. This defect may be related to the fact that AIDS victims have low levels of the hormone thymosin (secreted by the thymus gland). This hormone regulates and activates the T-lymphocytes.

Lymphocytes are specialized blood cells which are stored in the lymph glands and are given the responsibility for protecting us against all sorts of hazards and disease-producing substances. Lymphocytes are divided into two types: T-lymphocytes and B-lymphocytes.

T-lymphocytes, activated in the lymph gland, are located at the base of the neck near the throat. Healthy T-lymphocytes are active. When they are reduced in activity, or when the host (the body) is exposed to a foreign invasion or to a new invasion the body is not used to, the result is disease.

The second defense cell, the B-lymphocyte, is produced and sent into the bloodstream. These defense cells have chemicals called antibodies, which seek out foreign substances and destroy them. This is how vaccinations work.

What do these antibodies do? They clump all these foreign substances together and take them to the liver where they are detoxified and eliminated, and excreted out the kidneys—before they cause any harm.

There can be problems with the auto-immune system —over-activity and under-activity. The former is termed hypersensitivity, and the latter is reduced immunity. Hypersensitivity can be related to allergies—conditions of food, air, water, etc.—the environment.

Reduced immunity can result in poor wound healing, being extremely susceptible to infections, colds, etc.

AIDS is associated more with an UNDER-ACTIVE IMMUNE SYSTEM.

When these systems, the T- and B-lymphocytes, are working to their utmost capacity, they protect the body from foreign invaders. This is how the immune system functions.

According to Western, allopathic medicine, getting a disease is dependent upon three factors: (1) a portal of entry (how the pathogen gets into the body); (2) the virulence of that pathogen; (3) the host's immune response (how it protects the body and fights the pathogen).

The Natural Hygiene approach to disease is very different from the orthodox beliefs.

Scott J. Gregory and Bianca Leonardo, Harvey and Marilyn Diamond, authors of the best seller *Fit for Life*; Anthony Robbins, author of the best seller *Unlimited Power*; and T. C. Fry, president of the College of Life Science and editor of the magazine *Healthful Living*, all agree that the Natural Hygiene concept—which began in the 1800's by M.D.s who saw the light—is the correct one. In a nutshell:

Individuals do not "catch" diseases. After a person has committed innumerable crimes against his body, it gets to a point where it cannot take any more abuse. It tries to throw off the toxins in innumerable ways, such as sore throat, diarrhea, sweating, coughing, sneezing, fever, boils and cysts, etc. These are not symptoms of diseases; they are merely signs of the body's attempt to purge itself of excess poisons.

One could compare the body to a toilet which is clogged with waste or something that doesn't belong there. It overflows. To remedy the problem, the putrefaction in the toilet must first be broken up, dissolved, and then expelled. So with the body.

Specifically: abuses, overindulgences, dietary deficiencies, excesses of all kinds—a health-destroying lifestyle—creates toxemia from within. This leads to degenerative diseases such as AIDS.

Most important—this belief—that the FORCE IS OUT

THERE AND POWERFUL—AND WE ARE HELPLESS PAWNS—CAUSES US TO FEEL ABSOLVED FROM ANY RESPONSIBILITY! Thereby we bypass the help that we (with Nature's help) can give ourselves—control over our own bodies!

TAKE RESPONSIBILITY FOR YOUR OWN BODY —AND ITS STATE OF HEALTH! Every person must be willing to stand on his own two feet.

But you do not know what to do? THERE IS HELP —AND WE ARE TRYING TO SHOW YOU THE WAY —IN THIS BOOK.

"OPPORTUNISTIC INFECTIONS"

Infectious agents known as microbes swim daily throughout our bodies.

Microbes can reside in one's throat, mouth, gums, nose, and gastrointestinal tract.

These micro-organisms (i.e., bacteria, fungi, etc.) are a part of every human being's food and chemistry. Even if we die of causes other than infections, they eventually eat our physical remains. Only healthy cells, tissues and organs in our bodies can effectively defend us against infectious micro-organisms.

One of the most important defense mechanisms in the destruction of invading micro-organisms is the blood leukocyte (white blood cell). These special cells ingest microbes and render them harmless.

Before leukocytes can be manufactured in the body, there must be an optimum supply of amino acids, Vitamins A, C, B_1, B_2, B_{12}, biotin, niacinamide, pantothenic acid, and others, as well as a complete balance of all the minerals and trace elements.

If even a single amino acid is deficient or missing,

leukocyte production is diminished or may even cease.

It is essential to understand that infections will occur not because germs arbitrarily decide to attack our bodies. Rather, illness occurs because our nutritionally deficient, debilitated bodies permit these microbes to set up residence.

In short, an opportunistic microbe is an infectious agent that produces disease only when the circumstances are favorable.

Nutritional deficiencies can severely impair the integrity of a healthy immune system.

ABOUT CANDIDA ALBICANS

Candida Albicans is a yeast-related infection. Some of the symptoms include: headache, stomach upset, malabsorption, ringworm, athlete's foot, constipation, chronic diarrhea, depression, rectal itching, etc. The problems occur when there is an abnormal fungus yeast growth (that is normally controlled by ''friendly'' intestinal bacteria).

The yeast invades and colonizes the body's cells, tissues, and finally, the body. A strong, healthy immune system will contain Candida's growth.

When the fungi get out of hand and colonized, they produce toxic chemicals which attack the immune system, permitting the fungi to continue their tissue invasion and to cause more serious symptomatic disorders. The immune system has been challenged so often that it loses its ability to eradicate Candida.

For this reason, persons with AIDS should be taken off all yeasted and fermented products—wines, beer, alcohol, sugars, dried fruit (which is concentrated natural sugar), refined carbohydrates, including breads, cheese, sour cream, soy sauce, vinegar, mushrooms. Most ''B'' vitamins are derived from yeast. We must starve the yeast cells.

Most important, the body's weakened, nutritionally based immune system must be strengthened; this restores its proper function. We want to starve the yeast cell, but not the patient.

The AIDS patient should also swab the anus, rectum, genitalia, mouth, gums, and throat with a natural fungicide.

Please refer to the Treatment section, on the use of hydrogen peroxide. Immediate and significant results are being achieved with the use of this product.

A renowned medical doctor and acupuncturist who is using natural treatments, Dr. Luc De Schepper, states that "the disease of the '70s was hypoglycemia (low blood sugar). The disease of the '80s is Candida Albicans. Both are the same disease."

It has been claimed that one out of every three persons has the disease. Many authorities suggest that the use of antibiotics upsets the fine body balance.

Autopsies of AIDS fatalities reveal that most of them had colonized yeast infections in the body, in the form of thrush and Candida Albicans. The body is inundated with this yeast infection. The body cells cannot breathe. The body must be detoxified, as outlined in this book.

The Candida yeast infection can be present on the lips. Be careful who you kiss on the mouth. It is possible that one can get Candida by kissing. This important subject requires some research. And putting one's tongue in another's mouth—who knows what bacteria can be transferred? Candida is also present in the rectal and genital areas. One can even smell it; it has a strong, cheese-like smell. Is it also possible that one can develop Candida from reaming (anal licking) and oral copulation?

Saliva may contain disease bacteria; it should not be used to lubricate the penis before intercourse.

EXOGENOUS CAUSES
(PRODUCED FROM WITHOUT)

Stress

There are many sources of stress in our modern society.

1. Economics: financial problems, an undesirable job or lack of one; job competition; job insecurity, etc.

2. Pollution: air, water, food, sound (TV and other electronic media, traffic, airplanes).

3. Vaccinations: strong reactions; allergies.

4. Drugs: (legal and illegal); alcohol and tobacco.

5. Dental work: different, conflicting metals in the mouth that set up electrical charges; mercury poisoning; lack of preventive dentistry; neglect of teeth.

6. Allopathic intervention: cortisone injections, thyroid medications, estrogens, unnecessary surgery and drugs.

7. Lack of contact with nature and earth, with animals and children.

8. Lack of social grouping; loneliness, rejection; feeling useless. (The unemployed and homeless, and elderly, especially.)

9. Fear of being attacked (rape, robbery, etc.) especially in big cities.

10. Worry—about one's health, marriage, employment, business, etc.

11. Trendy styles (footwear—high-heeled shoes); tight-fitting garments; dyeing of hair, etc.

12. Synthetic materials—ubiquitous in our environment. Supersensitive reactions to artificial products (pesticides, herbicides, etc.). Plastic undergarments and other clothes, blankets, dry cleaning. Formaldehyde, etc., in building materials. Toxic chemicals in homes (over 100 toxic chemicals are used in the modern home today). Toxic chemicals in office buildings and factories—in the building materials, and used as cleaning products, etc. Other common toxic chemicals are used in everyday products, such as glue. These chemicals are absorbed either through the mucous membranes or the skin. They trigger chemical desensitization of the immune system, and cause behavioral disorders, mood swings, migraine headaches, allergies, epilepsy, depression, and ultimately, death.

13. Nutrition: marginal nutrition, vitamin deficiencies and excesses, can significantly affect your body's ability to properly handle drugs, environmental chemicals, and can influence your immunity to disease.

SUBSTANCES DELETERIOUS TO THE IMMUNE SYSTEM

TOBACCO, COFFEE, and ALCOHOL create an ADDICTION CYCLE. SUGAR and DRUGS are also addictive.

Alcohol:

The main problem with the use of alcohol is malnutrition. Nutritional deficiencies lead to alcoholism, predisposing conditions such as hypoglycemia, adrenal insufficiency, chronic fatigue, a craving for a ''lift'' (candies, snacks, soft drinks, all sugar products and caffeine).

Excessive drinking creates a vicious cycle by depleting

the body and leading to deficiencies in the B-vitamin complex, especially B_1 and B_6. Alcohol also depletes the body of zinc and magnesium. It washes the B vitamins out of the body; it creates a physical-psychological-social addiction and a reduced immune response. The advanced alcoholic suffers from liver and kidney damage. Cirrhosis of the liver leads to death.

The best substitutes for drinking alcohol are: glasses of fresh fruit juice; plenty of indoor and outdoor exercise that will improve circulation and general health and normalize the activity of the hypothalamus, the appetite center of the brain; plenty of rest; and a belief in a power greater than yourself. (The Alcoholics Anonymous program is excellent.)

Generally, most alcoholic beverages are processed with dangerous chemicals and preservatives. Nitroprussides have been proven to cause cancer; they are used in the manufacture of most beers.

Caffeine:

Caffeine is found in both coffee and tea.

Like alcohol, it washes out many nutrients, especially Vitamin C. It has a stimulating effect on the nervous system and is a drug—a poison to the body.

In coffee, there are chemical stabilizers, fresheners, color enhancers, artificial aroma ingredients; over 150 chemicals have been cited in commercial coffee.

If one drinks enough of it, it can produce premature ventricular contractions of the atrium (PVC's of the heart).

While working at U.C.L.A. (University of California, Los Angeles) Cardiac Care, I experienced working with night interns who were forced to stay up late at night to take care of patients, with no sleep. They kept themselves awake with coffee. At least three interns in one year were rushed to the emergency room with PVC's—they had overstimulated the heart. They had not had previous heart problems.

In Oriental medicine, it is taught that the taste of bitter stimulates the heart. Too much of that taste endangers it. We are not meant to eat many bitter foods. Most of the foods we get from Nature (fruits, vegetables, seeds, nuts) are sweet, and our tastebuds reject bitterness.

Why do people drink coffee?

People drink coffee because with cream and sugar, it tastes good, gives them a lift, "a caffeine high." The most dangerous aspect of coffee is that after the first cup, you don't remember how much you have drunk. With the coffee pot going all day in offices, factories and homes, people are not aware of how much they consume. Also, in work places, coffee breaks are social events, and the media associate "good times" with coffee drinking, alcohol and smoking. Thus they promote these habits; it is a brain-washing, a form of indoctrination. The health of the people suffers, because of Big Business wanting to sell its harmful products.

Small quantities of coffee benefit the body because the substance is a diuretic, but large quantites concentrate the toxins and wash nutrients out of the body. It is what is added to coffee that makes it so harmful. Coffee is highly concentrated and addictive.

Tannin:

Tannin, or tannic acid, is found in black and green teas, and is harmful. It is used in tanning and dyeing.

There is more caffeine in black tea than in coffee! But coffee seems to be more harmful, because of what the processors do to it. Commercial teas are not as heavily processed as coffee, but are still deleterious to the health.

Herbal teas are good alternatives. You will find them in health food stores.

Drugs:

In Oriental medicine, it is said that drugs of all kinds are the hardest substances to be gotten out of the body in a detoxification process. All drugs can cause harmful side effects. Most drugs interfere with normal enzyme and vitamin action in the body, causing derangement in the metabolism and vital body processes. Drugs destroy vital minerals and vitamins, and/or prevent their absorption. Many drugs damage the liver and kidneys, and can cause serious diseases, resulting in death. Drugs are physical irritants which weaken the body's immune system; they cause impotency, infertility, and birth defects.

Sugar:

Dr. Weston Price, a dentist in the early 1900's, discovered that primitive cultures thrived and were virtually free from diseases, including tooth decay, cancer and other chronic diseases. When the white man arrived with his sugar and processed foods, physical degeneration became rampant in a short time—within Dr. Price's lifetime. The natives developed crooked, decayed teeth, and degenerative diseases they had never had before the white man's arrival. Dr. Price was a pioneer in the study of how important nutrition is to good physical health, and the harmfulness of man-made foods.

In Oriental medicine, it is taught that the taste of sweet stimulates the spleen. An excess of sweet substances damages the bones and bone marrow. One of the causes of diabetes and arthritis is an excess of sugar.

''Refined white sugar drains out all the mineral salts of the blood, bones, and tissues,'' wrote the famous herbalist Jethro Kloss in his classic book *Back to Eden.*

Sugar cane, as found in Nature, is a good food. When a person sucks on a stalk of sugar cane, he is getting minerals from the sweet juice, and exercise for the gums. But after the sugar cane is processed (and lime is used in the processing, which leaches out the minerals), the end product, called refined white sugar, becomes a concentrated poison of no nutritional value. In fact, it is extremely harmful to the teeth and to the entire system. Entire books have been written on the harmfulness of sugar.

Tobacco

Tobacco causes an addiction brought about by certain physiological body dependencies which develop by prolonged usage. The addict's blood is poisoned and the poisons must remain high at all times. As the level of toxins drops down, he feels the urge to light up another cigarette, or to drink another cup of coffee, or to take some alcohol, to bring the toxin level up again. These are called cravings, and the addict has a physiological dependency as well as psychological cravings.

If nicotine is injected directly into the bloodstream in very minute amounts, it will kill; therefore, it is a poisonous drug in the body, as caffeine and alcohol are. Tobacco is a vasodilator and vasoconstrictor of the walls of the arteries and affects blood sugar levels and moods. Consequently, when people smoke they get a temporary sense of well-being, as with all other drugs. Smoking is also bad for the heart and lung tissues.

The only way physical and psychological dependencies can be broken is by CLEANSING THE BODY COM-

PLETELY OF ALL ACCUMULTATED POISONS, be they nicotine, caffeine, alcohol, sugar, or drugs.

LET US PURIFY THE BLOOD AND ALL THE CRAVINGS WILL CEASE!

The Story of the Coca Leaf and Cocaine

"In certain valleys between the mountains grows a plant called coca, which the Indians value more than gold and silver. The mystery of this plant of plants is that those who chew its leaves never feel cold, hunger or thirst."

—SPANISH DOCTOR WHO VISITED THE ANDES IN **1555**

In a television documentary, the tragic story of the coca leaf (from which cocaine is derived) was told. High up in the Andes Mountains, the common people chew this leaf.

They do not have enough food. The coca leaf stops hunger; it is an appetite suppressant. It also gives them great energy, and increases their ability to withstand cold. The coca leaf is an important part of their lives.

Commercial interests have changed this leaf to a drug. In the processing of the coca leaf, they have altered it, concentrating it, making a poison out of it.

Because of the tremendous amounts of money involved, the drug trade has brought crime—rape and murder—to the simple people of the Andes. These are the by-products of the great lust for cocaine and for money.

Bolivia is a very poor country. The people can scarcely feed themselves. But in the lowlands of Santa Cruz de la Sierra, and other underdeveloped backlands, is a booming $2 billion economy—based on coca, the scraggly plant from which pure cocaine is extracted.

U.S. drug enforcement agencies are struggling to cope with the flood of cocaine from Bolivia with little success.

More than half the cocaine that enters the United States comes from Bolivia. Apparently there is high-level corruption —governments involved in the international drug trade. Bolivia will not cooperate in stemming the tide, as the economy is "hooked on cocaine." And the peasants would rather grow coca than oranges and rice, which cannot match the profits of cocaine.

However, one peasant interviewed in the documentary said: *"The **coca leaf** is God's gift to us. But **cocaine** is of the devil and makes people crazy."*

In the Bible we read: "God hath made man upright, but they have sought out many inventions."

WHAT IS CAUSING MANKIND TO DESTROY ITSELF IN EVERY POSSIBLE WAY?

Cocaine is considered to be one of the most dangerous drugs of our time. THOSE WHO USE IT AND ABUSE IT (AND ANY USE IS ABUSE) ARE DAMAGING THEIR IMMUNE SYSTEMS.

THE HEART OF THE HEALING PROCESS

The Adrenal Gland

All stresses in life, whether physical, chemical, emotional or mental, put the adrenal glands to work. Sickness and disease also fall into these categories.

When the stresses are excessive and of long duration, the adrenals are overly taxed, and our energy-fire, stoked by our adrenals, is diminished. The adrenals are two small, thumb-sized glands located on top of the kidneys. When physical and mental stresses become excessive to this endocrine gland, our adrenal energy is diminished. The adrenals produce and secrete hormones directly into the blood, which help regulate a wide range of our body's normal functions, including the energy for healing, metabolic and sexual activity.

If we are threatened by a ferocious animal or see an imminent accident, or are pressured by a job that we *must* get done in too short a time, the adrenal glands pump life-saving adrenaline into our bloodstream, forcing us to move out of harm's way. If the adrenal glands are in a state of continuous overwork (which most are, since most of us live in cities with daily stresses), adrenal energy must be built up. To accomplish this, proper nutrition and reduction of stress are vital. Stimulants, such as sugar, caffeine, nicotine, drugs, alcohol and "pick-me-ups," should be eliminated. These stimulants directly affect the adrenal glands.

When one feels "down" and needs a "lift" he needs energy. How is he going to get it? What most people do is consume one or more addictive drugs or chemicals. This results in the adrenals being over-stimulated, and the body is put into a temporary high energy state. The initial result is a high level of sugar, alcohol or drugs in the bloodstream, which causes the pancreas to secrete insulin, and the rush of fuel is available to the cells. But then the negative happens.

The initial rapid pouring of detrimental substances into the bloodstream allows a profuse flow of insulin; then the blood sugar quickly disappears from the bloodstream into the muscles and liver.

THE RESULT IS: LOW BLOOD SUGAR. The consequences are: fatigue, anxiety, depression, headaches, and ill temper. Add a host of other symptoms and guess what results? A CRAVING FOR MORE QUICK ENERGY! So the person reaches for another candy bar, drink, cup of coffee, cigarette, drug—and he is in an addictive cycle.

MORE IMPORTANTLY, THE ENERGY FOR HEALING THAT YOU NEED FOR AIDS IS NOT MOBI-

LIZED AND USED! The weaker your adrenals get, the weaker your immune system gets, and you will be more vulnerable to all diseases.

Everyone must be educated as to ways of increasing energy without using stimulating chemicals like the above, which are not only addictive, but taxing to the adrenal glands.

YOU CAN CONQUER YOUR CRAVINGS. Rebuild your adrenal gland's energy, and CREATE A TRUE, NATURAL HIGH (ENERGY) FOR YOURSELF.

The first thing you must do is to break away from substances that hammer away at your adrenals. CLEAN YOUR BODY THOROUGHLY (using our methods), and stop taking addictive, over-stimulating substances that are very harmful to your health.

THE CRAVINGS WILL LEAVE WHEN YOUR BODY IS CLEAN.

DR. CACERES on DRUGS
as MAJOR CAUSE of AIDS

Dr. Cesar Caceres of Washington, D.C., has stated: "Drug use depresses the immune system. I first suspected this in 1982, and by October of '83, I had 12 people I could trace who had died of AIDS, so I put all their charts together and started going over them to see why *they* were dying. I looked at their backgrounds: they were all the same person! They had all been drug users for over five years."

We are quoting from the magazine *Christopher Street* (Issue 99). The article is: "You Think That Sex Causes AIDS? You've Been Had," by Ann Giudici Fettner.

"According to his calculations, based on figures from the Centers for Disease Control, Caceres maintains that 79% of those with AIDS in this country should be categorized as drug abusers. The remainder of cases may be categorized as Haitians, children, blood recipients, and that enigmatic group known as 'no known risk factor.'...

"Which drugs? 'In Washington,' Caceres says, 'it's been MDA, LSD, and amphetamines. MDA is a horrible drug that gives some people severe gastroenteritis, which can last for days. Another popular drug in D.C. is called 'blotter acid,' and from New York City they were importing crystal meth and 'Purple Haze.' Intravenous drugs aren't big here, and even cocaine wasn't that prevalent a couple of years ago. Washington's a surprisingly conservative town. But more coke is beginning to show up, along with more THC.

"I thought it odd that all those early deaths were among drug users, and it didn't hold for 100% of the cases, of course. It's dropped to between 80% and 90%—which it still is today....

"Reports are making the medical rounds that half of those with AIDS use as many as five street drugs in a year, that 93% smoke grass, 97% use poppers, around 68% take some form of amphetamine, and 70% take one or more drugs intravenously....

"Because information on drugs other than heroin isn't elicited by researchers, even physicians treating patients aren't aware of recreational drug use. This kind of information doesn't come out easily. You have to know the doctor won't give you the bad eye when you admit drug use."

METHAMPHETAMINE— "POOR MAN'S COCAINE"— INCREASING IN USE

Twenty years ago, methamphetamine was called "speed," and was popular in capsule form. Today it is usually produced as a crystalline white powder that is sniffed through the nose or mixed with water and taken intravenously. It is increasing in use. Its side effects range from hyperactivity to paranoia. Known on the street as "crank," it can be made almost anywhere, and the police are kept busy locating the illegal laboratories.

"It's rampant; it's all over the place. In the last year, we've really seen it mushroom," said Joe Doane, chief of the Bureau of Narcotics Enforcement in California. "I'd have to say we are a source state for other states."

Illicit labs even pose a threat to people who have never considered using such drugs, Doane noted. In addition to the explosive danger posed by ether and other chemicals, waste products and other toxic materials are often improperly stored. "Any way you shake this stuff, it spells nasty, dangerous and awful," added Doane.

William Pollin, director of the United States Institute on Drug Abuse, said: "We've gone through a period of approximately 20 years during which there was a dramatic increase in the use of drugs in this country. . . . If you get a 100 percent increase, that's epidemic. **In the area of drug abuse, WE HAD A 3,000 PERCENT INCREASE."**

FOUR

PREVENTION

Prevention of a disease is far preferable to trying to cure it. The common proverb has it this way: "An ounce of prevention is worth a pound of cure."

The best prevention is keeping one's cells healthy. But people generally don't think about their cells. The most important factor in keeping cells healthy and preventing AIDS is oxygen. When the body is clogged with toxic waste and polluted, the cells cannot breathe.

1. ABSTINENCE from sexual intercourse. In any sex-related disease, this is the best prevention.

Measures to help control lust are: eliminating meat and drugs from the lifestyle, and developing some spiritual pursuit, such as meditation. (We are reminded of the three-word command of St. Paul in the Bible: "Flee youthful lusts." Many people are now giving this precept serious thought, finding it is now related to the grave matter of life and death.)

If the individual finds abstinence impossible, then safety precautions should be used, such as:

2. A SINGLE PARTNER. It is recommended that one not engage in sex with multiple partners.

There is no evidence that AIDS spreads through shaking hands, sneezing, talking, or touching. Many doctors believe that anyone infected may be contagious for a long period of time, even though there are no symptoms. As a matter of fact, the infection may be present before the symptoms appear.

Deep kissing with heavy exchange of saliva has dangers. Who knows what poisons may be present in the saliva?

Women can also pass AIDS to their sex partners, but female-to-male transmission is not common (except with prostitutes), and the disease is virtually unknown among lesbians.

Avoid sexual relationships with high-risk people—male and female prostitutes, the promiscuous, etc.

3. USE CONDOMS (which will prevent the viral infection in the fluid from being transferred to the partner).

4. CLEANLINESS—washing the genitals both before and after intercourse, especially with germicidals. (Recommended: Herbal Septic, produced by NF Factor, and an Edgar Cayce formula called Glycothymoline, found in health food stores.)

More attention should be directed toward keeping one's hands clean and having clean facilities. Personal hygiene has been neglected, and now much attention should be paid to it.

Also—keep your body free from another's excretory wastes.

And remember: anal intercourse is the number one vehicle for transmission.

The alternative modes which are natural and holistic will be presented here and can be used as both prevention and treatment.

Ours is a clean country. We have more bathrooms per person or family than any other country in the world. But what is happening now is that, among certain groups, there is no respect for bodily fluids, and this is causing problems.

Better sanitation and personal hygiene, cleaner conditions and habits, would lessen the dangers of contagion from this and other diseases in the U.S. and elsewhere.

5. BLOOD TRANSFUSIONS: If one is necessary, know who the blood donor is. Demand this in the hospital. Refuse blood from foreign donors; ask to have blood from a member of your family or a friend who is healthy.

6. AVOID POSSIBLY CONTAMINATED NEEDLES from illegal drugs. **BETTER STILL, AVOID DRUGS ENTIRELY.**

THE THYMUS GLAND

The thymus acts as the filter for the glandular system, functioning like the liver. Its second use is to change negative thought patterns and speech to chemical secretions which are then filtered through the lymphoid tissue of the tonsils. The medical profession understands some of this, and today is not so often automatically removing the tonsils of children.

Because the thymus gland is both physical and psychological, a person with a normally functioning thymus is bubbling over, sparkling, and full of enthusiasm, with boundless energy and able to communicate optimistically to others. Small children are like this.

The thymus is situated in the upper part of the chest

cavity, along the trachea, and is a one-ounce glandular body considered to be a part of the lymphatic system. It is known to function in stress situations. Endocrine studies recognize a reciprocal relationship between the thymus and the sex glands. The thymus is known as a youth gland because after puberty, it shrinks in size.

As far back in history as 1902, a London physician named Foulerton was using thymus extract in the treatment of cancer. In humans and animals in which the thymus gland was removed or destroyed, there was a loss in the effectiveness of the immune mechanism which guarded the body against infection and cancerous growths.

Dramatic atrophy of the thymus gland can occur within a day of severe injury or sudden illness; millions of lymphocytes are destroyed and the thymus shrinks to half its size.

Dr. Lloyd W. Law, of the National Cancer Institute, found that thymus extract is essential in resisting cancer growth and development.

The more we can stimulate thymus activity throughout our lives, the greater will be our ability to ward off diseases like AIDS. (See the Treatment chapter.)

THE LYMPHATIC SYSTEM

The lymphatic system both feeds and cleans the entire organism. Most of the body receives nourishment directly from the lymphatic system, rather than from the blood. In fact, most of the cells of the body never come in direct contact with the blood.

The lymph nodes act as garbage collectors for the body. Most of the individuals with AIDS I have advised had painful, enlarged lymph nodes.

LYMPH: a colorless, odorless liquid which flows through the lymphatic vessels of the body. It bathes all body cells, collecting in tiny ducts, and lymphatic channels that wind near skin, muscles, bones, and organs throughout the body. It is an absorbent substance generated by the cells of the body which channels the lymphocytes to the blood. The blood, in turn, transports the waste to the lungs, kidneys, colon, skin, for elimination from the body.

Because of this, I recommend tissue cleaning by first cleansing the colon with chlorophyll and pure water solutions in high (very thorough) colonics or with a colemic board, to be explained later. After these, a hot, wet sauna should be used to cleanse the skin. The skin is one of the most powerful eliminating organs of the body.

If the lymph glands get plugged up by toxins to the point that they cannot move protein out of the system for a period of time, degeneration, disease, and death occur.[1]

Almost all tissues of the body, except a very few, have lymphatic channels that drain excess fluids from the interstitial spaces. Even these exceptions have minute channels through which the fluid can flow. Eventually, this fluid flows into the lymphatic vessels along the periphery of the tissue, or in the case of the brain, into the cerebral spinal fluid, and directly back into the blood.

It has been recently pointed out that many nutrients have positive effects in activating the immune system.[2]

To keep the lymphatic system clean, it is necessary to eat foods that are non-congesting. AVOID HIGHLY RE-FINED, CHEMICALIZED FOODS. In order to stop AIDS and preserve health, ONE MUST RETURN TO NATU-

1. Anthony, Catherine Panker, *Textbook of Anatomy and Physiology,* 7th edition, St. Louis, MO, Mosely & Co., 1967.

2. Salmon, J.W., and Berliner, H.S., *Why Contemporary Medicine is Failing,* American Journal of Acupuncture, Series 8, 1980, page 191.

RAL HEALTH LAWS, and use mild foods and healing herbs.

A number of herbs are particularly good for cleaning the lymphatic system—especially Poke Root, Golden Seal, Echinacea, and Cayenne. These foods can give a good balance of minerals and vitamins: vegetables, fruits, and their juices; seeds (some sprouted); grains, and very small quantities of animal by-products (milk, cheese, and eggs) —but not the flesh foods themselves. Use a wide variety of vegetables (mostly raw and steamed; frying is the poorest method of preparation). Fruits should be eaten raw, with rare exceptions.

A diet consisting of many sweets, meat, other animal products, and many refined, processed, overcooked foods will not heal the lymphatic system, but clog it further.

A new danger in food safety and purity has just arrived —the irradiation of foods. ''The powers that be'' are saying it will prevent food spoilage, and will not hurt us. But it is more likely to be the ultimate in cancer-causing substances in our lives. Americans need to investigate and protest this.

The three best ways to cleanse the lymphatic system are natural ones.

1. Deep Breathing. With every breath, the diaphragm moves, so do other muscles, the peripheral tissues, and the lymphatic vessels. Movement circulates lymphatic fluid.

2. The Kinesthetic. Bodily movement increases circulation. Best exercises are walking, swimming, and dancing.

3. Detoxification, as outlined in this book.

To CONQUER OR PREVENT AIDS and other degenerative diseases, PRACTICE ALL THE HEALTH PRINCIPLES EXPLAINED IN THIS BOOK.

FIVE

NATURAL TREATMENT— THE GREGORY METHOD

In the beginning of this century, we were healthiest nation in the world. Now we are the wealthiest, and the sickest. Why? There are many reasons. Now that most of the people in our country do not live the simple life on farms, but unnatural lives in the city, one must get knowledge in matters of health and well-being, and make extra efforts if one desires longevity with health, not sickness.

In AIDS, the body is unable to cope with conditions in which the cells are being slowly devastated by the sum of all wrong substances that are put into the system (drugs, alcohol, nicotine from tobacco, harmful food, etc.) plus poor environment (air, light, etc.), plus other persons' diseases.

In treatment, let us not deal with a disease, but rather with mistakes in lifestyles. Radical changes are required —from health-destroying habits to a health-building program. Thus, the ultimate road to a total elimination of AIDS is not finding a single cure (such as a vaccine), but rather, adopting a health plan which has a large scope—of both education and prevention. This will make the disease controllable.

STRENGTHENING THE IMMUNE SYSTEM OF AIDS PATIENTS

STEP ONE—HYDROTHERAPY. The patient, upon rising, takes a shower, first starting with warm water, gradually going to cold water, then back to warm water, and then ending with cold. Never apply cold water directly to the head—it is too much of a shock to the central nervous system.

Father Kneipp in Germany originated this method of treatment, and said that water is able to cure every form of disease, by dissolving the diseased matter and enabling it to be expelled from the body.

This water treatment has a special toning effect which rejuvenates and heals the entire system. It stimulates the circulation, and increases muscle tone and nerve force. It stimulates the entire glandular system, it improves the digestion and speeds up general metabolism.

Set the water on as high a force as possible. The higher the force the greater the stimulation, and greater therapeutic value.

After the shower, a quick, brisk rubbing with a coarse towel is in order. In Europe, showers like this are taken for several hours, resulting in greater health benefits.

STEP TWO—STIMULATING THE THYMUS, PHY-SICALLY. Imitate ''Tarzan of the Apes'' thusly: with your fist clenched, beat on your chest in the middle (see photo section). The beating stimulates the thymus function. Do this six or seven times, rapidly.

It is interesting to note that large apes and gorillas beat on their chests when they need strength—when in danger, or need aggressive behavior of any kind.

STEP THREE—DRY BRUSH MASSAGE. This is the next step, which takes only from five to ten minutes a day. Most health food stores have soft, plant fiber brushes with natural bristles; the brush is about the same size as the hand. It is long-handled so it can reach all parts of the body. The cost is approximately $2.00.

Do not use synthetic or nylon bristles; they are too sharp and can damage the skin. In the beginning, you should start with a brush that is less harsh and more gentle, until your skin becomes conditioned. Then you go to a coarser brush. The best time to brush is directly after your shower in the morning, and again before retiring.

The dry brushing basically is like a mini-acupuncture treatment—it stimulates the acupuncture points and meridians, unblocking stagnation and ridding the body of toxins by exfoliating dead skin cells, speeding up the circulation, rejuvenating the slowed-down cells. It increases cell metabolism. Accumulated waste products in the tissues are broken up—this process helps oxygenate the cells. Under ideal circumstances, the body cleanses itself automatically, without any effort on your part. It is a self-cleaning, self-protecting mechanism. Self-cleaning is performed by specially designed organs, glands, and transportation systems—the alimentary canal, kidneys, liver, lungs, skin, and mucous membranes of various cavities. But your largest eliminating organ is your skin. There are thousands of sweat glands which detoxify, regulate temperature, cleanse the blood and free the system from poisons.

The kidneys excrete toxins. Urine and sweat have almost the same chemical components. Uric acid, which is found in the urine, and excreted by the kidneys, is also found in large amounts in perspiration. When the skin is clogged, the liver and kidneys have to work harder to get rid of wastes. And the result is that the kidneys and liver become overworked, and eventually weaken or become diseased. The tissues become overloaded with toxins and wastes.

Benefits of the dry brush massage: It stimulates the circulation; it revitalizes and increases the eliminating capacity of your skin and throws toxins out of your skin; it keeps your pores open and helps lymphatic cleaning.

Most important, it helps relieve lymphatic clog. The brush should be washed with soap and water and put into the sunshine. When you brush, avoid irritation; don't brush infected or damaged parts of your body. Don't brush your face or private parts (they are too sensitive). You may brush your scalp. The combination of dry brush massage and hot-and-cold showers is an excellent way to stimulate and rejuvenate the glandular system.

How to Dry Brush Massage

Start with rotating circles on the bottom of one foot. Go up and down the legs and hips, then do the other foot and leg, then buttocks. The outside of the body is the YANG side, or stronger side; the inside of the leg area is the YIN side, and more sensitive.

Now, dry brush the arms, going down the front and up the back. Concentrate on any painful area. Do the chest and back; be gentle on the chest. The body and skin will glow. When you start, use small, short strokes, ending with large, sweeping strokes over the entire body.

STEP FOUR—ADRENAL MASSAGE. Now, the body is ready for adrenal massage (see picture section). Use a circular rotation motion with the two index fingers on the left and the right side of the navel. It is a rapid rotation motion. Sometimes the voice will even lower as male hormones are produced.

A warm drink of Taheebo (Pau D'Arco) Tea is suggested at this point. This tea has a strong anti-fungal action and anti-infectious properties that stimulate the immune function and improve digestion by destroying Candida Albicans.

Incidentally, if you think that we are giving you a lot of work to do FOR your body, just consider what you probably have been doing AGAINST your body, for a long time. What is needed now is for you to LOVE YOUR BODY! By this we mean—care for it, be good to it!

Now It Is Time for Breakfast and Supplementation

Please refer to Chapter 6 on Supernutrition and what to eat for breakfast.

Now It Is Time for Your Walk

You deserve a break now, so take a walk in the fresh air, swinging both arms. Be relaxed; do not carry anything.

(Are you wondering—When do I go to work? Listen, brother, THIS IS YOUR WORK NOW—GETTING WELL!)

STEP FIVE—LYMPHATIC CLEANING AND CO-LON IRRIGATION. A flat, fiberglass board that fits on your toilet, a five-gallon plastic bucket, and a small rectal tube is called a colemic apparatus.

The bucket is filled with pure water plus chlorophyll liquid, which you can buy at your local health food store. The proportions are: one eight-ounce bottle to five gallons of water. The colemic process is similar to an enema, except that you don't have to get up, and the water and waste material flow in and out by gravity. No pressure is created. The rectal tube does not have to be inserted very far, and is disposable after using; the morbid matter, waste, and toxins are gradually washed out and the chlorophyll is implanted. Dead cells and discarded tissue that have been accumulating in the colon (causing disease, premature aging, malabsorption) are loosened and expelled from the system.

As the water fills the lower abdomen, a slight finger pressure on hard areas expels water and toxins. Our systems, by way of the kidneys, bowels, skin and lungs, do all the eliminating, in a healthy individual. The alimentary canal and the bowels are the main road by which these toxins are thrown out of the body. Many toxins and wastes harden, encrust and remain in the colon, and reabsorb into the system, poisoning the whole body. Your body will try to get them out, particularly through the kidneys, which, as a result, become overloaded and damaged. This is why during a disease in which the body cannot eliminate wastes, the organs become overworked and fail, and death results.

The colemic cleansing process is a gradual one, and after the bowels are cleaned, the water loosens caked-up residues on the inside lining. The bacteria, mucus-ridden excrement is expelled into the toilet, where it belongs! Patience is necessary, because the body is not always ready to release its poisons all at once.

YOU MUST BE WILLING TO DO THIS—IN ORDER TO HEAL YOUR BODY!

There are many positive effects from colon cleansing.

One is that the lymphatics become unblocked, appetite is regained, absorption is greatly increased, mental abilities are improved, the eyes clear, one can work longer hours without fatigue, the disposition improves (toxins make one irritable, angry, sluggish, mean!)

And, of course, toxins make one sick. It is truly said that "death begins in the colon."

The people of the world are polluted within—and this causes the antagonisms and strife—because the internal toxins make people angry as well as sick.

This is so important that we wish to emphasize it: COLONICS AND COLEMICS NOT ONLY CLEANSE THE BODY BUT THE MIND! When the body is loaded with toxins (and everyone's is—unless they are cleaning the colon constantly), the person becomes irritable and angry—the toxins affect the mind.

We, the authors, have noticed this effect in ourselves. Contrariwise, after a colon cleansing, one becomes kind, amiable, loving—as well as getting a big surge of energy!

WE MUST NOT ONLY EAT PROPERLY BUT AS-SIMILATE AND ELIMINATE!

Mere emptying the bowels on the toilet is not enough! YOU HAVE A CHOICE OF A COLEMIC (at home, just described—you do the process yourself, or with the help of a family member)—or a COLONIC—where you go to the office of a health practitioner who gives colonics.

Just one of either will not do the job! The first few times you have the colonic or colemic (the latter is more thorough), you will notice that the process helps soften and carry away intestinal debris. But the real cleaning comes after this intestinal putrefaction is removed, and one actually gets down to the mucus in the lining of the intestines.

Research has demonstrated that the colon has reflex points that affect the organs—so the physical process of the water entering and being expelled has a toning effect

—not only on the intestinal system, but also on stimulating the various organs.

A well-developed tissue-cleaning system is very good to help overcome pain in all parts of the body.

In working to overcome a serious degenerative disease such as AIDS, it is recommended that the treatment be ongoing and constantly applied. Every day is best, for the first week. If the patient drops in energy suddenly, the process must be halted.

It should be understood that this treatment is not a cure-all, but an important step in the detoxification program.

THIS DETOXIFICATION PROGRAM IS VERY POWERFUL. TREMENDOUS HEALING CAN BE ACCOMPLISHED!

Some precautions must be taken. Because of the elimination of toxins, your body becomes weak. You must rest and take supplementation after a colonic treatment. It is best to retire after a colonic or colemic.

Not all the toxins are expelled. Some of them go back into the system. Therefore, if it is at all possible, go into a wet sauna—the same or the next day. Those toxins which are in the circulatory system are pushed out through the skin.

BENEFITS OF COLONICS AND COLEMICS

After a colonic or colemic (or series of them), you can expect:

1. Your eyes to lighten in color;
2. Sores on the body to heal more quickly;
3. Increased energy;
4. Clearer thinking;
5. A general feeling of well-being;

6. The skin will glow with radiance;
7. Joint and back pain will lessen;
8. Darker skin on the genitals and rectum will lighten (the dark flesh indicates blood stagnation);
9. The appetite will increase;
10. An extended stomach will be reduced, with repeated treatments;
11. Much Candida Albicans and bacteria will be washed out of the colon;
12. You will achieve a more youthful appearance.

To maintain their health, beauty and youthfulness, actresses Gloria Swanson and Mae West did intestinal cleaning daily. They both lived to an advanced age with health and youthfulness. Intestinal cleaning is one of the best secrets for health and longevity. Friends tell me (Gregory) that I "look ten years younger" after a colemic.

Ventrux-Acido and minerals (Body Toddy) should be taken after a colemic, to replace the nutrients which may have been washed out. The small intestine manufactures many nutrients, especially B-vitamins. It is important to keep it clean.

It is advisable, if you have low blood sugar, to use chromium (hypoallergenic) after a colonic/colemic. Chromium helps regulate blood sugar levels.

A colonic or colemic can temporarily make you feel weak for these reasons: a tremendous amount of toxins are eliminated from the body. When the body is healing, energy is consumed.

It is advisable to take your colemic before retiring, so the body can rest and heal.

STEP SIX—THE SAUNA. Steam cleaning your body is similar to steam cleaning your car! Many people do not take as good care of their bodies as they do their cars!

Parmenides, ancient Greek philosopher and physician, said: "Give me a chance to create fever, and I will cure any disease." Naturally, when a body's resistance is low, it reacts by producing fever. It is a part of the body's defense mechanism. But when the body is in an extreme weakened state, artificially induced fever can be used. The high temperature speeds up metabolism and energies and the fever itself fights infection. This procedure is not only effective for the common cold, but degenerative diseases as well.

There are many ways to induce fever. Medical doctors use drugs to induce fever—but the sauna is a more natural approach, which we recommend. It stimulates the body's defense naturally; there is less stress on the body, and there are no side effects, as with drugs. But do not use the sauna if you have heart problems or high blood pressure.

Artifically induced fever has been used by natural doctors for acute infection, disease, arthritis, skin disorders and cancer, to name only a few. The length of time and the temperature of the sauna should be monitored. A professional should do this.

The skin is called "the third kidney"; it has tremendous eliminating properties. Some European nations—Finland, for example—are more aware of this valuable therapy than the U.S. This process is also called "The Finnish Steam Bath."

As with the colemic or colonic, the sauna stimulates vital organs and glands, and increases their activity. Basically, through profuse sweating, toxins are eliminated and organs stimulated.

Steps in a Sauna

First and foremost, the sauna must be wet and not dry. It must be warm enough for profuse sweating but not uncomfortable (should be relaxing, not painfully hot).

Because individuals have different heat tolerances, we cannot specify here what temperature the steam should be, nor how long to stay.

In Finland, dry heat is not used—only wet saunas.

HERE IS THE PROCESS: One wraps oneself in a towel and sits or reclines. Shortly, perspiration will commence.

At this time, massage painful areas of your body. The pores will be open. Now, to facilitate the eliminating process, the dead skin can be rubbed away with the fingers or a brush. The more dead skin is removed, the more the pores will be opened.

Now you leave the steam room. Do not take a cold shower now; let the body cool down naturally. Lie down and rest, at least half an hour. Now you get up and rinse in lukewarm water, scrubbing the skin again. Finally, you can use very cold water and use a rough towel to dry yourself.

THAT IS THE END OF YOUR SAUNA—UNTIL NEXT TIME. GO AT LEAST TWICE A WEEK.

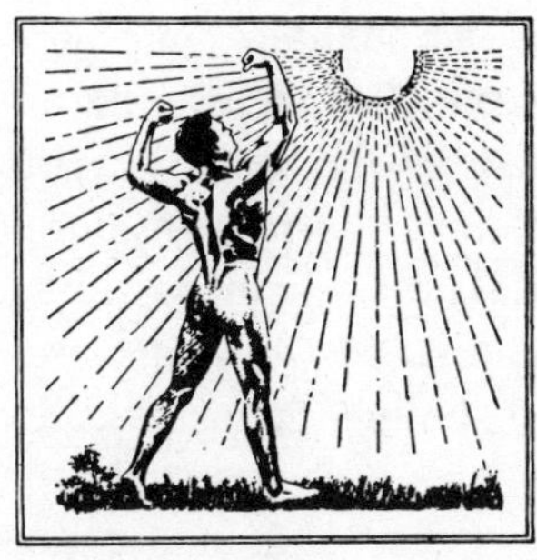

STEP SEVEN—SUNSHINE THERAPY. The sunshine therapy does not start for one week. The reason is this: Sunshine stimulates the production of T-lymphocytes, and the present ones are infected, so we don't want to produce more of those.

Before the AIDS patient can utilize the benefits of sunshine, he must be producing normal lymphocytes. This is accomplished by lymphatic cleaning through nutrition, specific herbs, and other modes of detoxification.

According to Zane R. Kime, M.D., in his book *Sunlight Could Save Your Life*:

"Sunshine aids in maintaining man's constant war against disease.

"The sun aids by destroying the germs in man's environment before they enter the body. Sunlight effectively kills germs in the air, purifies water, destroys bacteria on exposed surfaces including the skin, and produces antibacterial agents on the skin from the oils present there.

"The sun aids by increasing the resistance of the individual. Sunlight increases the production of and stimulates the activity of the lymphocytes, neutrophils (part of the red blood system), and other cells of the immune system. These cells in turn produce more antibodies (gamma globulin) and interferon to circulate throughout the body. The net effect is that the individual's defenses against disease are greatly strengthened."

Stress produces adrenaline, and adrenaline produces cyclic adenosine monophosphate, a harmful chemical substance that circulates in the cells.

Coffee, tea, nicotine, and polyunsaturated fats also contain this chemical. The sunlight destroys this agent.

Sunlight is beneficial for most diseases. Dr. A. Rollier of Switzerland used sunlight therapeutically in his mountaintop hospital in the Alps with tremendous success—leading to the recovery of tuberculosis and cancer patients. They were treated under timed and controlled conditions and were never allowed to burn.

In the case of AIDS, after detoxification, the sunshine is a great therapeutic agent in building interferon and prostaglandins (hormone-like substances that are produced from a certain essential, unsaturated, fatty acid called linoleic acid).

In his book, Dr. Kime reveals how sunlight, properly employed, can lower high blood pressure, lower high blood sugar, decrease total body cholesterol, strengthen a physical fitness program, increase the body's resistance to infection, and prevent some of the chronic degenerative diseases which commonly plague western civilization.

Sunlight increases the oxidation of the blood. An increase of oxygen to the tissues promotes healing of a variety of infectious diseases. Oxygen promotes healing by directly strengthening the immune system; therefore, it is beneficial for the AIDS patient.

RULES FOR THE SUNBATHER

1. Exposure must be gradual. Start the first day with a minimum of time—no more than 20 minutes.

2. Time of day: The best times, when the sun is not so hot, are: before 11 A.M., and after 3 P.M. (depending upon your location, time of year, etc.). The angle of the sun rays is most propitious between 3:00 and 4:00 P.M.

3. It is totally individual. Some people can spend hours in the sunshine without burning, while others burn very readily. Sunlight does not readily penetrate dark skin.

4. Drugs, cosmetics and soaps can sensitize the skin so that a burn develops.

5. Don't overheat. If it feels too hot, get out of the sun. But sometimes, with ocean breezes, one cannot tell one is burning. So—time yourself. You could wear white clothes—the sunlight will penetrate. Wear sun hats to protect the face. And—nude bathing is best, if possible.

6. Never use sun screens or lotions: Many, including the so-called natural ones, can cause cancer.

These sunscreening agents block out therapeutic effects of the sunshine.

It is important to expose all orifices of the body to the natural sunlight at an approximate 45° angle (usually between the hours of 3:00 to 4:00 P.M.)

The sunlight is of great benefit in many ways to the body.

First, open your mouth wide; the entire oral mucous membrane is given exposure. The eyes are kept closed.

The genitalia are next exposed. Exposure does not have to be long; five to ten minutes are sufficient. The cheeks of the posterior are spread and the rectum is allowed to see sunlight.

In 1877, two scientists found by accident that natural light can kill bacteria. A section of the electromagnetic spectrum was proven to have tremendous antibacterial action (in 1892, by Marshal Ward). Many scientists, such as Arloing, Polerino, Duclaux, Koch, Moment, Henri, Chemelewsky and Dieudonne, used sunlight for killing bacteria.

Nobel Prize winner Niels Finsen used sunlight in the treatment of tuberculosis patients. Sunlight was used before the invention of antibiotics. Some of the diseases that sunlight cured were: viral pneumonia, bronchial asthma, blood poisoning, peritonitis, mumps, and many other infections. In 1976, L. D. Heding found that *ultraviolet light has the potential of inactivating and destroying cancer pathogens.*

Dr. Stanley Folkow, professor of microbiology and genetics at the University of Washington School of Medicine, states that "all the presently available data strongly suggest that perhaps as soon as the next decade we are going to see serious antibiotic resistance among all groups of medically important pathogens."

The AIDS pathogen might be one of these.

The significance of this is: Antibiotics will not be able to cope with our current pathogens (scientists are alarmed about this). Therefore, we should again turn to natural methods, such as using sunshine or ultraviolet light.

Sunlight therapy was used extensively years ago, and was growing in favor, as the results were encouraging. With the discovery of antibiotics, sunlight therapy was neglected. Let us return to discover this marvel of Nature, and use sunshine as a natural therapeutic agent.

Sunlight is a tremendous agent for destroying bacteria-sensitive germs. Here are some common germs that sunlight or ultraviolet light can kill:

The anthrax bacillus
The plague coccobacillus
Streptococcus
The tubercle bacillus
The cholera bacillus
Staphylococcus
The colon bacillus
The dysentery bacillus

SUNLIGHT INHIBITS CANCER BY STIMULATING THE IMMUNE SYSTEM and increasing the immune efficiency and increasing oxygen to the tissue. Cancer cells cannot thrive in a high-oxygen environment.

It is suggested as a protection, before going into the sunshine, that you follow a diet containing plenty of foods high in anti-oxidants, which are Vitamin C, E, A-Carotene, but low in animal fat and without refined oils.

Anti-oxidants are free radical fighters. Free radicals cause mutations in the DNA and hence aging, cancer, etc.

Dr. Alan Cantwell, M.D., a scientific researcher in the field of cancer microbiology, and author of the book *A.I.D.S., The Mystery and the Solution* (1984), states that the most probable cause of AIDS is a bacterial infectious agent, not a virus, and there is a certain relationship between AIDS and cancer.

STEP EIGHT—OCEAN WATER THERAPY. Ocean water has therapeutic value in the treatment of disease. Many naturally occurring minerals can penetrate the skin. The water should be clean and a comfortable temperature for the patient. Sea water has been analyzed by chemists, who have found that there are similar minerals and salts in our blood serum and in the sea.

The German physician Heinz Graupner wrote in his book *Adventure in Healing* that "sea water is one of the last medicaments (healing applications) provided by Nature to have found its place in modern medicine" (at least in Europe).

DRINKING WATER

Humanity cannot live without water. We have often asked the question, "Why must our bodily wastes be channeled into our water system?" Our water is precious and everything possible must be done to save it from pollution —preventing industrial dumping of chemicals, etc. In order to purify water for drinking, strong chemicals must be used, which are harmful and possibly are carcinogenic.

Therefore, use only pure water, such as bottled water, for drinking and cooking. Glass bottles are preferred to plastic containers, because PVC (polyvinyl chlorides), chemical resins, and plasticizers leach out of the plastic into the water. Many persons believe that boiling tap water purifies it. But not all the germs are killed and certainly the ammonia and chlorine are not totally boiled off. So only use pure, fresh water. There are very good companies that deliver clean, fresh, pure water to your home. Investigate the choices in your area for the following reasons. Firstly, there are few or no laws controlling bottle sterilization. Secondly, there are no laws governing the purity and safety of water used by water companies.

SUPPLEMENTATION— GENERAL INFORMATION

Supplementation should be used to fill nutritional gaps produced by faulty eating habits and when the body's resistance is so low that absorption is a problem.

We do not recommend additional supplementation on a daily basis for a healthy body. Body chemistry balances are very delicate. Unless you are absolutely sure (and who is?) of your deficiencics, supplements can upset the balance of your body's chemistry.

Our bodies, when healthy, make what is needed. Many ''B'' vitamins are produced in a healthy intestine. The mere taking of these ''B'' vitamins can throw off the balance. Our bodies have developed the ability, or always had the ability, to biologically transmute or change elements to whatever is needed. Our bodies can and do, according to the theory of biological transmutation, change magnesium to iron in the body, mica to calcium, etc.

However, vitamin supplementing does have a place

when used therapeutically. It can be of tremendous help as a prevention measure in fighting disease and assisting the body to speed up its recovery. Vitamins do not heal; the body does.

The main reason that herbs work is because of their vitamin content—in the perfect balance that Nature created. However, a knowledge of herbs and their properties is needed; some have poisonous components.

Vitamins can correct some deficiencies and help conditions caused by them. This is achieved by the vitamins acting as a metabolic catalyst—turning on body activities.

In large doses, vitamins protect a variety of bodily functions by stimulating, rather than acting as a catalyst—speeding up or slowing down reactions.

Today our foods are loaded with chemicals and toxins; they are processed, refined, saturated with pesticides, insecticides, fall-out, radiation, etc. Vegetables and fruits are picked unripe—this makes them without nutritional value at least, or else poisonous. To get adequate nutrition from commercial foods today is a real problem—in fact, one might say, it is impossible.

Many individuals are lacking vitamins, minerals, enzymes and proteins due to fast foods loaded with chemicals, residues, foods that come from depleted and unfertile soils. ''Big business'' keeps using heavy preservatives and long periods of cold storage. Today, nutritionally inferior and poisoned foods cause many nutritional deficiencies and even disease. The prime reason for supplementation is to fill gaps. If possible, buy your food in a Co-op (much is naturally grown), or better yet, grow your own (if possible). Some health food stores have organic produce, and in some cities, there are ''Farmers' Days'' when small farmers bring their produce to market.

As a rule, most supplements should be taken with meals. They work best that way. Some vitamins are antagonistic. For example: Vitamin E should not be taken with iron. These two vitamins are antagonistic, and should be taken at least eight hours apart.

Here are some things that interfere with vitamin absorption: Smoking destroys Vitamin C; aspirins and other drugs and alcohol interfere with the absorption of "B" vitamins; rancid foods and chlorinated water interfere with Vitamin E absorption.

Physical body disorders and mental stress can interfere with vitamin utilization.

Please do not buy your vitamins in a drugstore. Their quality is inferior.

Natural vitamins do not occur in nature by themselves. Over 28 factors have been found in Vitamin C alone. New vitamins are discovered daily in foods. Our knowledge of vitamins is not complete. Therefore supplementation should be used only for short periods in acute conditions or when there is severe deficiency.

Rules In Using Supplements

Vitamins should be natural and hypoallergenic, especially with a suppressed immune function (see section on allergies). Most hypoallergenic vitamins are synthetic; try to find natural ones.

The vitamins must be fresh and not stale (they are dated). Vitamins should be rotated, to give the body a rest from the same substance. Vitamins should have co-factors to help absorption. (Examples: "B" vitamins with co-factors; Superoxide Dismutase with the enzyme catalase, for proper absorption.)

Some supplementation is better taken on an empty stomach but most are better absorbed with meals. Vitamin C is a diuretic and washes minerals out of the system; therefore, it should be taken with minerals. We recommend minerals in the form of aspertates—they are less apt to cause allergies.

When suffering from a serious disease, it is unwise to attempt self-treatment with vitamins, minerals, or any other way, but it is advisable to consult a doctor who is nutritionally oriented.

The most exciting new information relating to nutrition that improves immunity is the work on dietary oils and their impact on immune functions. It has been found that people who are on highly saturated animal-fat diets or diets rich in partially hydrogenated vegetable oils, or those who cut almost all fat out of their diets for long periods of time, may have a suppressed immune system due to an essential fatty acid deficiency.

Again, BALANCE IS ESSENTIAL!

HERBS

DETOXIFYING HERBS—Used as a tea infusion:
  Echinacea; Chickweed; Burdock
CLEANSING HERBS: Golden Seal; Yellow Dock; Black
  Walnut; Yarrow; Pau D'Arco
HERBS THAT BUILD THE IMMUNE FUNCTION: Red
  Clover; Chaparral; Buckthorn; Licorice Root; Poke Root;
  Sho Wo Che
HERBS THAT STRENGTHEN THE GLANDULAR SYS-
  TEM: Saw Palmetto; Lobelia; Mullein

(Take 1½ teaspoons of any one or combinations, in boiling water.)

SUPPLEMENTATION FOR THE
AIDS PATIENT

* Explained in greater detail in this chapter
* * * Indicates greater importance

* * * VITAMIN A, in the form of Beta-Carotene (see p. 86). (*Country Life; Solgar*)
VITAMIN B's—with co-factors, including B_{12} and high potency B_6, hypoallergenic (no corn, soy, wheat or yeast). See ISO-B.

* * * VITAMIN C—with minerals; hypoallergenic. Source: Sago palm (*Dr. Steven Levine*)
VITAMIN D—from sunshine (See Appendix)

* VITAMIN E—Mycel. (See page 63.)

* EVENING PRIMROSE OIL—liquid drops. Can be applied to Kaposi's sarcoma. (Most reliable: *Aubrey Organics*)

* THYMOTROPIC HORMONE with raw thymus. Includes vitamins, minerals, enzymes. (*Enzyomatic Therapy*)

* CERNILTON FLOWER POLLEN (*Cernitin-America*)

* DENTIE (*Chico San*)

* GLYCOTHYMOLINE (*Edgar Cayce Formula*)

* SUPEROXIDE DISMUTASE (S.O.D.) (*Organik*)

* ZINC PICOLINATE PLUS—Picolinic Acid and Pancreatic Tissue; enhances absorption. B_6 (*Ethical Nutrients*)

* MUCOPOLYSACCHARIDES

* GLUATHIONINE

* L-LYSINE (*Solgar*)

* PROTEASE ENZYMES

* * * HYDROGEN PEROXIDE
       (Food Grade, undiluted, 35%)
    * VITAMIN B_{15}—Pangamic Acid (D.M.G.)
      Oxygenates the cells; increases body's resistance
      (*Country Life*)
      AL 721 (Egg Lecithin)
      CO-ENZYME Q-10 (*Immune Modulator*)
    * EXTRA-ENERGY ENZYMES (*Biotec Foods*)
    * VENTRUX-ACIDO (Acidophilus culture—
        non-dairy) (*Cernitin-America*)
    * PROTEOLYTIC ENZYMES (anti-inflammation)
        (*Nature's Plus*)
    * RED CLOVER
    * CHAPARRAL
* * * MEYER'S LAPACHOL (Pau d'Arco—Tincture or
        Elixir)
* * * ASTRAGALUS (herb for the immune system)
* * * CAPRICIN
* * * BODY TODDY (*Rockland Corp.*)
      ECHINACEA TINCTURE (*Enzyomatic Therapy*)
      PANCREATIC ENZYME
* * * NUCALMAG (Calcium Magnesium Butyrate)
* * * SOMARIN (*Dr. Henry Mee*)
* * * C-KIN (*Ishii Enterprises*)
* * * ALOE VERA (freshly pressed)
      FREE-FORM AMINO ACIDS—AMINO
        HEALTH (*Integrated Health, Green Label, L.*)
        (See p. 20)
        NUTROX (very potent anti-oxidant) (*Integrated
        Health*)
    * ULTRA CHOLINE (contains Manganese, B_6 and
      other minerals) (*Integrated Health*) Available from
      health professionals only.
      ISO-B. (hypoallergenic vitamins) (*Integrated Health*)

* IMMUNE TONICS Nos. 1 & 2 (Chinese Herbal Tincture Preparation) (*KW Botanicals*)
* CARNIVORA (from the Venus Flytrap plant)
* FEVER FEW (fol Chrysanthemum parthenium)
  LIQUID LIVER
  LIVA-TOX (*All 3, Enzyomatic Therapy*)
* * * BULGARICUM—I.B.

(If the reader has difficulty finding these natural health supplements, he may write: "Supplements," P.O. Box 1222, Santa Monica, CA 90406.)

SUPPLEMENTATION—
IN-DEPTH DESCRIPTIONS

* VITAMIN C—In large quantities, administered orally, 20 or more grams per day, just to the point of diarrhea. Powder is best because it dissolves easily in liquid. Buffered and hypoallergenic. Take on an empty stomach. Dietetically speaking, use vegetables especially high in Vitamin C and Beta-Carotene. These foods include: dark green and deep yellow vegetables, citrus fruits (preferably organic), the members of the cabbage family. Refer to the chart in the Appendix ("Foods High in Essential Nutrients").

* VITAMIN E—According to research conducted by Dr. Cheryl F. Nochels (University of Colorado), animals were given Vitamin E equivalent to four to five times the FDA requirement. Results: improvement in activity of the T-cells was three to five times that in response to bacteria, viruses, and cancer cells than the immune systems of animals supplemented with Vitamin E at lower levels.

* EVENING PRIMROSE OIL. This actually is the oil from the evening primrose flower; the product is mixed with Vitamin E. It provides us with a vital nutritional component and is one of the few sources, other than mother's milk, of GLA (gamma-linolenic acid). This substance is needed for the body to make a family of hormone-like compounds that control every organ in the body. These compounds especially affect the heart, circulation, skin, and DEFENSE MECHANISMS AGAINST DISEASE. Anyone having a deficiency of GLA will also have a shortage of PGs (prostaglandins). It is not a drug. At one time it was thought that GLA could be made in the body from essential fatty acids from linolenic acid. It has been recently proven that many bodies do not manufacture this compound, especially sick bodies.

GAMMA-LINOLENIC ACID, found in Evening Primrose Oil, STIMULATES THE T-CELLS OF THE IMMUNE SYSTEM AND HELPS CELLS TO REVERT BACK TO THEIR NORMAL STATE.

The compound called PGE is required for the T-cells or T-lymphocytes of the immune system to attack pathogens. In fact, PGE plays a major role in the regulation of the thymus gland, as well as T-cell function. Thus, Evening Primrose Oil is required in optimum quantities to maintain an optimum immune system. Reversing these cells back to their normal size is a new approach.

The Evening Primrose Oil does no harm to normal tissue, as radiation, chemotherapy, and drugs do.

Very little attention has been paid to the possibility of normalizing abnormal cells. This is largely because the dominant theme of research into AIDS today is that the disease is brought about by irreversible and uncontrollable mutations within the nuclear DNA.

Evening Primrose Oil makes the cell more receptive to Vitamin C when both are used together.

About the American Indian and His Use of Herbs

The American Indian knew of the medicinal properties of Evening Primrose Oil, and gave it to the Pilgrims. It was taken to England, and there called "The King's Cure-All." In the U.S. there are a number of species with different names.

An interesting sidelight is this: When the American settlers pushed back the Indian on this continent, they decimated his race. They put the remnants of a people onto reservations, where often the men degenerated into idlers and alcoholics; the white man's liquor had been introduced to the reservations. A tragic result for our own people and our own time is that the INDIAN'S HERBAL CULTURE WAS ALSO DESTROYED. The succeeding generations on this continent have accepted Western medicine—almost totally based on chemical drugs and surgery.

We admit that in the field of surgery, marvels are being done. But in the area of diseases, little is being done in prevention—in educating the people how to take care of their health. In cures, there is such an over-dependence on drugs—with such vast monies involved—that this leads to DRUG DESPOTISM. The serious side effects of drugs definitely point to looking for another healing modality, and we present it here.

* THYMOTROPIC, with raw thymus (by Enzyomatic Therapy). It has been discovered that the thymus gland secretes important hormones, the most important being thymosin. Giving the patient raw thymus extract concentrate plus nutritional supplementation increases the level of thymus function and T-cell production. The most important nutrients to build the immune function are: Vitamin C, Vitamin E, minerals, zinc, and hormones like thymosin.

* CERNILTON FLOWER POLLEN from Sweden. A fermented flower pollen concentrate, developed by A. B. Cernelle of Engleholm, Sweden, the pollen is of specific interest.

The deoxyribosides in the product can penetrate a cell wall and can be absorbed by the cell.

Cernilton has the ability to stimulate interferon production. Studies have shown that the pollen increases the body's immunity to illness and stimulates and rejuvenates gland activity by building up the body's restorative powers.

The Cernelle company of Sweden has been studying pollen from flowers since 1950. Pollen is one of the richest and most complete foods in Nature. It contains amino acids, vitamins, minerals, enzymes, plant hormones, unsaturated fatty acids, deoxyribosides for the production of DNA and RNA, and many other essential biofactors. (See list, p. 177.)

Pollen is the male germ cell of the plant kingdom. *Flower pollen, not bee pollen, is the richest and most complete food in nature.* Flower pollen contains 20 percent protein, all the water-soluble vitamins (with the exception of B_{12}), and a rich supply of minerals, trace elements, enzymes and co-enzymes. There are also sterines and traces of steroids.

* DENTIE reduces contagion in the throat and oral cavity. Made from the calyx portion of the eggplant, it is charred, and sea salt is added. This black powder is painted on the back of the oral cavity. It is also excellent for brushing the teeth and gums.

In Oriental medicine, Dentie is said to have the strongest of the "yin" (the eggplant) combined with the strongest of the "yang" (sea salt). It is an ancient folk remedy used by Oriental peoples for centuries.

* GLYCOTHYMOLINE (an Edgar Cayce formula). This

is a natural cleanser and disinfectant, mouthwash and gargle. The rectum and the genital areas can be washed with this preparation. It can be used before and after sexual intercourse. It is also used as an expectorant.

* SUPEROXIDE DISMUTASE. "S.O.D." is a copper-bearing enzyme which triggers the body to its proper function. It is best taken sublingually (under the tongue). S.O.D. fights free radicals, which are unstable, unpaired, swirling electrons. Free radicals have the ability to penetrate a cell, causing changes in the DNA, which produces mutation. Free radicals create:

1. lipofusion (brown age pigment—cellular "garbage" below the skin)
2. cross linkage for enzymes (RNA and antigens)
3. mutations
4. chromosomal breaks
5. cancer

These free radicals attack cells which are damaged, resulting in the tissue losing its integrity. S.O.D. neutralizes and prevents some of the tissue damage. S.O.D., combined with catalase, an enzyme, inhibits rancification of lipids or fats in the cells. These slow down and deteriorate the cell. S.O.D. performs quite a number of other beneficial functions within the body. S.O.D. is a prime agent for keeping ourselves in a balanced metabolic state. It does this by helping the body rebuild the worn-out cells.

S.O.D. is reported to be universal in all plants which grow in oxygen; the greener the plant, the more S.O.D.

Chlorophyll, the green in all vegetation, releases oxygen. Eat unsprayed kale, collard greens and broccoli. All these are natural high sources of S.O.D.

S.O.D., with catalase, is one of the best known free

radical scavengers. Sprouted grains and seeds are found to be higher in S.O.D. than cooked. S.O.D., first used in veterinary medicine, is now being successfully used for treatment of inflammation.

Nuclear fallout, radium contamination from watches, gold jewelry, effects from radium and cobalt treatments in cancer patients, microwave cooking, excessive X-rays used by dentists and the medical profession, could develop into radiation poisoning in the body. S.O.D. products have been used to counteract the effects of all these man-made menaces.

Recommended: Organik Q-10 (Co-enzyme 10) S.O.D. plus catalase.

* ZINC—It has been recognized that nutritional factors in several diseased states contribute to zinc deficiency in man. Weight loss, severe recurrent infections, or immune disorders may be related to zinc deficiency. Studies show that dietary amounts of zinc in the United States may be so low as to cause health problems. The mineral zinc is not easily assimilated. Zinc picolinate is a zinc supplement designed to increase zinc absorption. (*Ethical Nutrients*.) Dosage: for proper maintenance of the immune system, between 15 and 30 milligrams per day. Zinc is important in activating the immune system but it must be in balance with the trace element copper. Zinc increases sperm count, it decreases the level of ammonia in the body, it promotes wound healing, increases appetite, improves the skin condition and improves the sense of taste and dark adaptation.

* MUCOPOLYSACCHARIDES help to glue cells together, lubricate joints and play a major role in the structural integrity of the body tissues that are responsible for connective tissue form. Mucopolysaccharides are involved in the transferring of electrolytes and nutrients through the cell wall. Crustaceans (lobsters, shrimps, crabs, clams,

mussels, etc.) are the best source of mucopolysaccharides. These foods also have a high quantity of RNA.

* GLUATHIONINE is a water-soluble amino acid used as an anti-oxidant which detoxifies (harmful) peroxides. Toxification levels are decreased. Another free radical fighter.

* L-LYSINE is a natural free-form amino acid that has a powerful anti-viral effect. Even a single shift of one amino acid can dramatically change body chemistry.

* PROTEASE ENZYMES. These split or break down proteins into polypeptides and peptides such as trypsin, bromelain, papain, which stimulate the formation of blast cells, which are the early developmental immune system cells. These are a type of white blood cell derived from the thymus.

* * * HYDROGEN PEROXIDE—A common substance with "magical" powers, whose significance is unrecognized or neglected.

There are over one thousand research papers today on hydrogen peroxide. Most of this research has been done at the Mayo Clinic. Yet, you will not find hydrogen peroxide mentioned in the Medical Desk Reference.

We live in an ocean of micro-organisms, each one seeking out its own little habitat in our bodies—from the tops of our heads to the bottoms of our toes. We can control or eliminate them from our bodies by drinking a simple solution of hydrogen peroxide!

Hydrogen peroxide is H_2O_2—water plus another molecule of oxygen.

It does more than just bubble. It is an antiseptic and infection fighter.

McGraw-Hill's *Encyclopedia of Science*, Fifth Edition, states that hydrogen peroxide exists in rain and snow, mountains and streams. How does it get there? It gets there from the ozone layer. Sunlight and the ultraviolet rays split the O_2 molecule. If not destroyed by pollution, the ozone reaches the ground. The hydrogen peroxide gets into our fruits and vegetables. It is a by-product of the photosynthesis process.

Hydrogen peroxide is not as unstable as believed. If you take a 3% solution of hydrogen peroxide and boil it, and check it for the liberation of O_2, the O_2 will still be present. It is not easily destroyed.

Human mother's milk, and especially colostrum, the "first milk," contains a high percentage of hydrogen peroxide; that could possibly be where we get our immunity. But how many babies are breast fed? Ever since commercial formulas were developed, and pushed on new mothers in the hospitals, very few (although there is a new trend among some young mothers to return to breast feeding).

Lancet, the renowned British medical journal, states that hydrogen peroxide has been used successfully with malaria patients. It has been used in many other ways, also—as an oxygen source at Cape Canaveral for the astronauts; as a preservative in products (food grade)—it triples the shelf life of many foods; aloe vera gel has naturally occurring hydrogen peroxide, and is used to heal wounds and burns.

In Europe, hydrogen peroxide is added to drinking water to purify it, instead of the chlorine and ammonia we use, because ozone has 5,000 times more killing power on bacteria than chlorine and ammonia. So why do we not use it, too?

At Lourdes, France, the water was tested and found to contain hydrogen peroxide. So—it is more than people's faith that is curing them at Lourdes!

The T-lymphocytes engulf and secrete chemicals that kill foreign cells. These two very important substances

—hydrogen peroxide and super oxide—are both reactive forms of oxygen. These materials are lethal to foreign bodies. Hence, they are given during treatment of AIDS.

AIDS is caused by a pathogen that cannot survive more than five minutes outside the body. Why? The germ is anaerobic: it cannot live in a high-oxygen environment. When hydrogen peroxide is taken into the body, it raises the oxygen level, and oxygenates the cells.

Dr. George Sperti, a medical researcher, is connected with the St. Thomas Institute, in Cincinnati, Ohio. He has over 23 patents, including two called Preparation H and Aspergum. For 14 months in the Cincinnati, Ohio, Cancer Center, **he conducted experiments on cancerous mice. In 30 to 60 days, 90% recovered, when treated with hydrogen peroxide in their drinking water. The tumors went into remission!**

When hydrogen peroxide is put into the system, it enters the bloodstream; there it seeks out the microorganisms and destroys them.

Scientists at the University of Iowa, University of Wisconsin, and Wabash College, Crawfordsville, Indiana, hypothesized that hydrogen peroxide is the ultimate cause of normal cell division.

We believe that the deficiency of hydrogen peroxide production increases an individual's susceptibility to infection.

Microorganisms themselves possess an electrical charge. When one suspends these organisms in an aqueous solution on an electrical plate, they will gravitate toward the positive charge. The hydrogen peroxide is short an electron on its outer orbit, and will accept an electron to complete its outer orbit.

The result of electrons being taken away from microorganisms is dead matter.

Hydrogen peroxide taken orally has been researched by Dr. Edward Carl Rosenow of the Mayo Clinic. Pathogens invade, attack cells, building cocoons around the stricken cells, cutting off blood supply and nutrition, causing only the infected cells to live, as in cancer and AIDS. O_2 increases the elimination of toxins. O_1 in ozone or hydrogen peroxide kills the infection.

Hydrogen peroxide, taken internally, must be without preservatives or stabilizers.

Dr. Otto Warburg (twice a Nobel laureate) states that "cancer cannot live in a high oxygen environment."

Dr. Rosenow took germ cells and fed them different foods and put them in a different environment; he got a different disease. When the food and environments were changed back to the original, the original disease resulted.

Conclusion: Specific germs live and multiply in specific environments. If the environment is changed, the germ will either leave or be destroyed.

If you do not believe this—the benefits of hydrogen peroxide—feed it to your pets and plants. They will thrive on it, and you will have first-hand evidence.

Recommended dosage is one ounce hydrogen peroxide (3 percent solution) to five ounces of pure water.

* VITAMIN B_{15}—Pangamic Acid—and DMG (Pure N, N-Dimethylglycine) are all one and the same substance. Natural sources are: root vegetables and whole grains. It increases the flow of oxygen to the body; it increases the hemoglobin (red blood cell) count, and takes ammonia out of the brain and the liver and tremendously benefits the immune system, by keeping the anaerobic and aerobic bacteria in check. Sublingual use (under tongue).

* EXTRA ENERGY ENZYMES—scientifically grown, biologically active, wheat sprout culture containing trace enzymes. Included is Superoxide Dismutase ("S.O.D.") and catalase. Vegetarian, hypoallergenic. (Biotec Foods, Honolulu.)

* VENTRUX-ACIDO—a product from Switzerland that helps unclog the digestive system. This product contains 75 million non-dairy lactic acid-producing bacteria in each small capsule. The product contributes to better digestion and assimilation of nutrients. The viable bacteria are: *Streptococcus faeclum* strain live bacteria. Recommended dosage, two to four small capsules per day.

* PROTEOLYTIC ENZYMES. These substances (ascorbic acid, quercetin, and bromelain) have been demonstrated to be significantly effective anti-inflammation agents. Here is a naturopathic approach to inflammation for the AIDS patient.

* RED CLOVER. A healing herb, usually combined in formula with other herbs; also builds the immune function and has special blood-cleansing properties. Used in a formula as part of the Hoxsey cancer treatment.

* CHAPARRAL—an herb that makes available minerals in the body where the cells need to be rebuilt.

* * * MEYER'S LAPACHOL, from a tree in Argentina which is most unusual. It lives in tropical forests where bacteria and fungi thrive, yet the tree is free from most parasites. The provincial Indians—since Inca days—have used the inner bark of the tree to combat internal and external infections.

This South American tree is called Ipe roxo and Pau d' Arco in Brazil, and Taheebo in Bolivia. The Lapacho tree of Argentina, with light-lavender flowers, is two to three times more effective than the dark red Brazilian tree or the yellow-flowering Bolivian Taheebo tree.

Dr. Theodore Meyer discovered the tree in Argentina, and now grows the trees on his wilderness plantations there, 100% organically, ecologically, without any chemicals.

The active ingredient in the inner bark of this tree is

called Lapachol. It is effective in combating gram positive, an acid-fast bacteria and fungus. Topically, it can be applied to sores and lesions with much benefit.

Quinones, alkaloids developed from plants, have many anti-cancer properties, and Lapachol has a full range of quinones.

According to Oriental medicine, Lapachol seems to work on the liver energy to advantage.

The Meyer Lapachol Elixir is the pure extract from the tree, and is recommended over other similar products.

* * * ASTRAGALUS. This is the Chinese herb that best builds and strengthens the immune system. Modern researchers are testing this herb to learn why it is so beneficial for the immune system. It works better than any other herb. Where there is no hope in Western medicine, herbs can be successfully used.

* * * CAPRICIN—a time-released fungicide. It eliminates unfriendly fungi without destroying the patient's friendly flora. It is important to note that the Candida Albicans fungus is able to penetrate deep into the convolutions of the intestinal tract. Capricin, being a lipid solution, is able to penetrate the cellular membrane, eliminating both the surface and inter-cellular Candida.

Dosage: 12 capsules per day with meals, for six months, tapering off slowly.

* * * BODY TODDY. A full spectrum of more than 103 minerals in liquid that replaces mineral loss in our bodies, caused by depletion in the soil and environmental pollution. This product is easily assimilable and nourishes the body with these needed nutrients. Body Toddy can be taken regularly. It is not affected by stomach acids or the digestive process, as are pills.

* * * NUCALMAG. This product contains butyric acid,

magnesium and calcium. Most food allergies and sensitivities are gone in 14 days when using this product. It is suited for the AIDS patient because it boosts the immune function. It has fungicidal activity, helps the body to produce its own short-chain fatty acids, and heals the gastro-intestinal membranes from Candidiasis damage.

* * * SOMARIN. Henry Mee, Ph.D., is using this product to improve lymphocyte profiles in AIDS and ARC patients.

Mushrooms and higher fungal compounds which have natural chemical activities are being used as a natural therapy. Somarin induces and improves helper-suppressor ratios, increases helper cell counts, and normalizes lymphocyte mitogen stimulation. No toxic side effects of this therapy are noted.

* * * C-KIN is derived from an aqueous extract of the fruit body of *Lentinus edodes mycelia* (LEM), or Shiitake, an edible Japanese mushroom—a popular food in several Far East countries. It is cultured on a solid medium of bagasse and rice bran. This product is a polysaccharide extract which has anti-tumor, anti-carcinogenic, antibiotic, anti-bacterial, and anti-fungal properties, and natural interferon inducers.

Also called Lentinan, it has immuno-pharmacological agents considered to be an effective defense against lowered immune status. Medical benefits of edible fungi remain still largely unexplored. This product can be used to strengthen the internal organs' activities, regardless of health status, and also alleviate exhaustion due to overwork and lowered resistance. Japanese experiments, on both humans and animals, have shown that this product potentiates host resistance, and it should be used more in this country.

The Shiitake mushroom is an outstanding nutrient source

of B-vitamins, manganese, magnesium, calcium, pro-vitamin D, L-Lysine. The Shiitake mushroom is an outstanding interferon-inducer, but because of the hard-cell membrane of its cap, much of it goes through the human gastro-intestinal system undigested.

Dr. Iizuka has solved this problem by creating a freeze-dried extract made from the mycelia (the spores or seeds of the vegetative portion of the thallus or head of a fungus), which feed on themselves and break down and absorb the hard membrane.

C-KIN is made from the mycelia, which are more potent than the mushroom itself, because the hard membrane is dissolved. One gram of C-KIN is equal to eating 1200 grams of fresh Shiitake mushrooms.

C-KIN overcomes collagen disorders and strengthens the immune system. This product has been used success-fully for disorders including cancer, leukemia, liver malfuntions, herpes, ulcers, hypertension, gout, kidney stones, acute allergies, arthritis, acne, hangovers, and many others. It stimulates the immune system itself and does not hurt healthy cells or have side effects.

* * * ALOE VERA, freshly squeezed. Aloe Vera is a succulent plant, the juice of which is used for healing wounds and burns. The main feature is a high oxygen content. It also contains allointin, a cleansing and prophy-lactic compound. It gives energy, heals damaged mucosae, and seems to reduce some lymphatic swellings. The juice is taken internally.

* ULTRA CHOLINE takes cholesterol from the cells and allows no transfer of toxins to other cells. At the Universi-ty of California at Davis, research is being done on Ultra Choline as related to AIDS.

* IMMUNE TONICS 1 & 2. These contain approximately 20 Chinese herbs that stimulate the immune system and clean lymphatic obstructions. They are immuno-stimulant glandular tonics which also tone the liver and kidneys. They are resolvents; they systematically and locally improve the immuno-deficient syndrome, reduce toxicity and inflammation in the body.

* CARNIVORA is the extract from the Venus Flytrap plant. It has 22 different gene-repair substances. Dr. Hans Nieper of West Germany has used it successfully in cancer and multiple sclerosis.

* * * BULGARICUM—I.B. *(from Lacto Bacillus Bulgaris)*. It activates the immune system; aids in the production of white blood cells; regenerates tissues; helps produce these important substances: ribonucleic acid, proteins, alpha amino acids. Aids longevity. Used as an anti-cancer preparation; tested on 100 oncologic (cancer) patients and clinical remissions recorded; all had good results. From *Observations on the Therapeutic Effect of the Anti-Cancer Preparation from Bacillus Bulgaris.*

SIX

SUPERNUTRITION FOR THE AIDS PATIENT AND OTHERS

Eating should be pleasurable; our food should be both delicious and wholesome. Everyone at the table needs to be in a cheerful mood, as this aids digestion. Let the food be attractively served.

AIDS patients have weakened digestive systems and so, at first, their food should be prepared in a blender and a juicer. They should eat blended salads (raw, blended vegetables) and freshly squeezed juices from organic fruits; also, pureed fruits and seed milks. THIS IS VERY IMPORTANT; there is much wholesome nutrition in these foods. THEY ARE LIFE SAVERS. We are advising *not that these foods be added to the regular diet* the AIDS patient has been on—*but that these foods be substituted for it.*

The diet we recommend is not any *one* strict diet (e.g.,

macrobiotic, or vegan, or totally raw, or a "Natural Hygiene" diet, etc.) It is made up of FOODS THAT HEAL. In this dietary consideration, we selected foods that do not create adverse reactions, and are easily absorbed, assimilated, and digested.

Our foods do not stress the immune system. We state that the body needs change. For example: cabbage, kale, cauliflower and Brussels sprouts are all in the mustard family. Foods in the same family have similar nutritional values. Eating too much of the same or similar food gives the body too much of the same nutrient. Because something is good does not mean that more of it is better.

Upon rising, the AIDS patient should take no food until two hours later.

(THE PEOPLE WHO LIVE THE LONGEST EARN THEIR BREAKFAST WITH EXERCISE—we are told by a number of prominent doctors in the natural health field. They have a relaxed lifestyle, with tranquillity, and usually a vegetarian diet—or with very little animal protein. They get fresh air, pure water, lots of exercise, have meaningful work, and truly loving relationships. They do not abuse their bodies in the ways that many city people do. They naturally include "The Seven Essentials of Health" [fresh air; pure food; water; exercise; sunshine; sleep and rest; positive mental attitude and a spiritual life]. Such people do not suffer from the chronic degenerative diseases that afflict many people who do not live by these precepts.)

The AIDS patient should drink the following juices: fresh blueberry juice or other berry juice (according to the season); carrot juice, freshly squeezed; grape juice, from fresh, preferably organic Concord grapes. Do not use bottled juices. By law, all bottled juices must be pasteurized, so these are boiled, filtered, and often have preservatives added. The nutritional value of the juice is gone; it is devitalized. Some of these juices are mere sugary water.

Do not use the frozen juice concentrates: It is believed that after the producers spray the oranges, they use them whole for the frozen orange juice. Rotten oranges could be used; we'll never know. Also, do not use the synthetic juices, called "as good as orange juice." They are no such thing—they are mere chemicals in the guise of orange juice.

THE FRESH JUICES AND FRUITS HELP TO BUILD THE RED BLOOD CELLS, AND IMPROVE THE CLEANSING FUNCTIONS OF THE GLANDS.

Figs help to feed the hormonal system; if they are dried, they should be soaked in pure water. Watermelon also cleanses the glands, but it should be eaten only during its natural season, the summertime. The watermelon's "meat" inside should be very red in color. Watermelon, as all melons, should be eaten by itself, not with other foods. This is one of the laws of proper food combining. Make a meal of the melon alone.

RAW OR COOKED FOODS?

Although many leaders in the natural health movement recommend raw foods as being superior to cooked, there are some foods not suited to the human stomach in their raw state. These are better cooked: potatoes and beets and other root vegetables (excepting carrots); grains (unless sprouted); asparagus; broccoli; cauliflower; eggplant; the squash family; beans.

The human system cannot possibly assimilate and digest these foods raw, because the starch molecule must be broken down or dextrinized by the use of heat. Raw starch is indigestible. Bananas should be very ripe (with spots);

otherwise, they are pure starch; one might as well eat a raw potato.

Fruits should be eaten in season, be ripe and organic for maximum nutrition.

Some devotees of fruit try to live on them alone. But fruits cannot sustain the body in superior health, exclusively.

City people who try to live on fruits from the supermarket (unripe and sprayed) will be seriously malnourished.

Even people in the tropics, who have an abundance of ripe, organic fruits, do not try to live on them alone. One sees that they intuitively cultivate grains and vegetables, for a BALANCED DIET.

In general, foods that are palatable raw should be eaten in that form. Foods not suitable to the human stomach raw are better cooked. (To steam vegetables is far superior than to fry or boil them.)

We do not recommend peanuts in any form. They are not nuts, but are in the pea family—often infected with a yellow fungus. In processing, they are often roasted, salted or sugared.

Cooked foods are much more readily digested and more easily absorbed, but many of the enzymes are destroyed in cooking, it is believed.

Amylase, one of the digestive enzymes that the body itself produces, initiates the breakdown of carbohydrates; this process begins in the mouth.

Some foods, when cooked, become toxic. For example: spinach produces oxalates, which rob calcium from your body, and cause stones. It is best to use spinach raw in salads.

Whole grains are wonderful foods; yet, they contain phytic acid, which destroys and stops calcium absorption, when it builds up in the body. So—don't overuse grains. Also, being carbohydrates, they produce heat in the body, and too many grains produce too much heat.

Three great secrets to health and long life are: small quantities of food, a great variety, and rotation of foods. Do not eat too much of any one food. The cells like variety! We do not want foods to become obnoxious to the system. What is good for your body today may have a different chemical reaction tomorrow! This is why wonderful Nature gave us such a variety of foods!

One who engages in hard physical labor needs stronger foods, and more quantity.

Everything in our universe is in a state of continuous change—the seasons, the environment, the activity, whether it be physical or mental.

In order for man to thrive, he must also make changes.

MORE DETAILS ON THE DIET

Most foods should be eaten in their natural state. The emphasis should be on raw vegetables, especially the green leafy vegetables, plus fruits (fresh, never canned), nuts (must be fresh, not rancid), and seeds: sunflower, pumpkin, and sesame.

Grains may be sprouted or cooked. Breads are not recommended, nor are the cold, boxed cereals. The best grains for cooking are millet, buckwheat, barley and brown rice.

A moderate amount of easily digested protein should be eaten, mostly of plant origin, including vegetables and grains.

Raw, unheated, unsalted cottage cheese, from high-quality, unpasteurized milk, can also be used.

Raw milk and milk products can be used if your body tolerates them well. How do you know if you tolerate milk well? If, upon rising, you have no congestion in the nose,

A DIFFERENT LIGHT BOOKSTORE
489 CASTRO (BETWEEN MARKET AND 18TH)
SAN FRANCISCO, CA 94114
415. 431-0891
OPEN DAILY 10-11 . TO MIDNIGHT FRI & SA

47611   B 04/11/92 4:02

14347   1 CONQUERING AIDS 12.95   12.95

             1 SUB-TOTAL   12.95
             TAX   1.10
             TOTAL   14.05
             Cash -CLERKS
             AMT TENDERED   20.05

             CHANGE DUE   6.00

happy springtime from a different light
Sorry: NO CASH REFUNDS store credit only

no swollen face, no skin irritation, or any kind of allergic reactions, or stomach upset, you are tolerating milk.

Some allergic reactions called "dysregulation" affect over half the population, making them sensitive to certain chemicals or foods that result in malfunction of the immune system. In a true allergy, the body's immune system triggers a defense reaction, producing dramatic effects. Some people's throats swell when they eat peanut butter, mushrooms, or other foods. Depression can also occur.

One woman (as stated by Dr. John Crayton, Associate Professor at the University of Chicago Medical School), had severe depression and mood swings when given corn extracts. She acted strangely, could barely open her eyes or her mouth. Tremendous improvement was obtained with the use of rotation diets, avoiding the foods that caused the allergy.

This example shows immune changes and suggests not a typical food allergy, but the body trying to neutralize toxins. It does this by producing antibodies.

With AIDS, the body is also trying to produce antibodies. This is why AIDS patients have digestive disturbances—their immune system is overworked.

Variety is very important. The worst thing we can do, nutritionally, is to eat the same food, day after day. The human body gets tired of the same nutrients. Pity the poor people in places such as Ethiopa and India, where they feel fortunate to have one food only, such as rice. This is why they are so unhealthy, and is related to why they are so backward and in poverty. (Of course, it is a vicious circle—the poverty also causes them to lack the proper foods.)

With AIDS, or any other disease, to drastically change your diet suddenly is detrimental. The body is trying to heal itself, and you throw it out of balance when you change the diet suddenly and drastically. Make changes gradually! Everyone is an individual, and all needs are different.

There are social differences among people; ethnic differences (with different food customs); environmental differences (hot and cold climates, with different soils); and occupational differences (people needing different daily caloric totals)—all these are important differences among people.

So we must learn to listen to the body and to its needs. The body does not like drastic changes, especially when it is in its healing state. One does not go from a meat diet to a vegetarian diet overnight. One must work at it, and do it gradually.

RULES IN EATING

1. Refrain from overeating at any meal. Leave the table only 3/4 full—in other words, before a feeling of surfeit sets in.

2. Always go outside after a meal. Reason: the body requires plenty of oxygen to assimilate food, especially proteins and starches.

3. Take slow outdoor walks from half an hour to one hour—before and after meals. This habit adds years to your life, because the exercise helps the food to digest.

4. Eat only when you are hungry. Hunger is indicated by a watering mouth and throat sensation. Nausea, headaches, addictive cravings, stomach disturbance are not symptoms of hunger. One should abstain from eating until hunger returns.

5. Chew your food well. Digestion begins in the mouth,

and the saliva is the first digestive secretion. The more you chew, the better your digestion will be. The food should be masticated well until it is liquefied, before being swallowed. If you have trouble doing this, you can put a small piece of raw carrot or celery in your mouth with the other food.

6. Do not eat when in pain, anger, a worried state, or have any other emotional upset.

7. Keep meals simple for easy digestion.

8. Soak dried fruits at least overnight, in heated, pure water. Make sure they have no sulfur dioxide or other preservatives or colorings.

9. Use pure vegetable oils (no commercial corn oils). You need cold-pressed oils or olive oil (extra virgin quality). These oils should be used as they are—in salad dressings, etc.—NOT HEATED!

10. Eat foods grown in the region where you live, for the most part. Every food has its season and location. Avoid foods that are picked green, gassed, preserved and shipped long distances. Eat more raw foods in the summer, more cooked foods in the winter. Seek out organic foods without pesticide sprays, embalming compounds, etc.

NUTRITIONAL ASPECTS: VITAMIN SUPPLEMENTATION

Many nutrients have positive effects on activating the immune system. A number of water-soluble and fat-soluble vitamins, as well as minerals and proteins, directly affect and activate the immune system.

VITAMIN B_6 deficiency depresses B- and T-lymphocyte functions and seems to accompany Vitamin B_{12} and folic acid deficiency. Of the water-soluble vitamins, Vitamin C is the most important. Vitamin C has been shown to play a very important role in activating T-lymphocytes and the Vitamin C content of white blood cells, which usually can become depleted during violent infection, stress, and pregnancy. Vitamin C supplements taken almost to the point of diarrhea—5,000 to 10,000 units per day—have been found to activate T-lymphocytes.

Fat-soluble vitamins and minerals to improve the immune system are:

BETA-CAROTENE: A pigment found in orange and red vegetables and fruits. It has been shown in human studies to be a potential protecting agent against smoking. In cases of induced lung cancer in laboratory animals, levels of Beta-Carotene intake of 10,000 to 30,000 units per day caused them to recover. One of the major benefits of using Beta-Carotene rather than Vitamin A is that there appears to be no toxicity from the Beta-Carotene, while toxicity symptoms from Vitamin A include hair loss, headaches, dryness of mucous membrane, skin problems, and digestive disorders, as well as increased liver damage. Vitamin E, another fat-soluble vitamin, has also been shown to have a beneficial effect upon the immune system. Both Vitamin A and E deficiency can depress the immune system, affecting one's general resistance to disease. If too much Vitamin E is given, suppression of the immune system occurs. Recommended dosage: 100–600 units is best per day for the immune system.

TRACE MINERALS also play an important role in activating the immune system. Iron deficiency is the nutritional deficiency that has been targeted by the U.S. Department of Agriculture as the most prevalent in U.S. society. This deficiency is also known to lead to immune suppression, as is the case with many other of the trace elements.

However, if a little is good, much more is not necessarily better. The optimum daily dose of iron is between 15 and 30 milligrams per day.

Zinc is another mineral that has a powerful effect on the immune system. The level of zinc required for proper maintenance of the immune fumction is between 15 and 30 milligrams per day.

Selenium and magnesium also have been shown to be important in activating the immune system. When the body is in a low, depleted state, sick and run-down, supplementation is suggested for a short period of time, because foods do not carry adequately high levels of these nutrients. Deficiency of selenium, along with Vitamin E deficiency, can greatly increase the risk of infection and may increase the susceptibility to AIDS and cancer. Selenium requirements can vary from between 100 to 300 micrograms per day; organic selenium is better than inorganic, the best source being selenite or selenate.

Magnesium depletion may lead to decreased function of the thymus gland—the gland that activates T-lymphocyte function. The average magnesium intake should be about 400 to 600 milligrams daily.

PROTEINS AND FATS: Dietary protein is another class of important nutrients which stabilize immune function. Protein which does not have the right balance of amino acids, such as incomplete vegetable protein, or heat-rendered animal protein, can result in impaired immunity, which increases the risk of low resistance and susceptibility to disease. For example, fad weight-loss diets for extended periods of time, a vegetarian diet with daily protein intake that is inappropriate to the particular body's needs, or the inability to assimilate or digest protein correctly—all can lead to infection.

Eating lower on the food chain (plant foods instead of

animal foods) is less dangerous in our polluted world. Animal protein can be toxic to a healing body. Most of us suffer from protein excesses.

Dr. Paavo Airola, nutritionist, points out in his book *How to Get Well*, that:

"Dr. Ph. Schwarz, of Frankfurt University, in Germany, and Dr. Ralph Bircher, a famous biochemist from Zurich, Switzerland, report that the aging process is triggered by *amyloid*, a by-product of protein metabolism, which is deposited in all the connective tissues and causes tissue and organ degeneration—thus leading to premature aging. This explains why people who traditionally eat low protein diets—Hunzakuts in Pakistan, Bulgarians, Russian Caucasians, Yucatan Indians, East Indian Todas—also have the highest life expectancy in the world—90 to 100 years! And why the people who live on high animal protein diets, such as Eskimos, Greenlanders, Laplanders, Russian Kurgis tribes, etc., have the lowest life expectancy in the world—30 to 40 years. Americans lead the industrialized world in per capita meat consumption—and they also are in 21st place in life expectancy among industrialized nations!

"Recently, Dr. Willard J. Visek, of Cornell University, implicated a high protein diet in the development of cancer. *Ammonia*, which is produced in great amounts as the by-product of meat metabolism, is highly carcinogenic and can cause cancer development. A high protein diet also breaks down the pancreas and lowers resistance to cancer, as well as contributes to the development of diabetes.

"These are just a few examples of recent research and overwhelming scientific evidence which show that a high animal protein diet is *a very dangerous course to follow*.

"Not only animal proteins but *all* proteins should be consumed in moderation. Excessive protein consumption, even if from such sources as milk or concentrated protein powders of vegetable origin, can be dangerous.''

ALL EXCESSES CREATE AN IMBALANCE.

WHAT IS ADEQUATE PROTEIN?

We are all unique. Genetics, daily activity, one's physical size and metabolism, one's constitution, custom—all affect dietary protein needs. Generally, men need more protein than women. Again—balance is the most important element.

It has been our general experience that most diseases come from excesses rather than deficiencies. We have listed in the Appendix some symptoms of both deficiencies and excesses in protein consumption.

If the individual does not create and maintain balance in his body, Nature will!

An example of how a person corrects imbalance is this: When a person runs, he sweats, thus releasing and excreting toxic wastes from the system. He may think he is running for exercise, to lose weight, etc.—but the real reason is that he must make balance in his system. His body is urging him to do this.

Persons also drink large quantities of water after heavy salt consumption, to adjust balance in the body; some also drink large quantities of alcohol to help the digestion of fat and protein.

Europeans, especially Scandinavians, take hot sauna baths to open the pores of the skin to rid the body of excess salt, fat and toxic wastes. These groups of people eat much salted cheese and fish—which create excess metabolic wastes.

The skin is a great detoxification organ, comparable to

the kidneys. Drug addicts have been known to get a drug reaction by tasting their sweat.

The best example of Nature making balance is sickness and death. Eating too much salt causes puffiness under the eyes, painful joints, high blood pressure, heart problems or kidney failure, the end result being death.

Grains, vegetables, seeds, fruits, are the easiest to balance. After a heavy meat meal most individuals feel they need a hot fudge sundae or other sugary confection to balance out the meat. Oriental medicine calls this balance "yin" and "yang"—the meat being yang, the sweet dessert being yin. We know these laws through intuition, but sometimes forget.

On a hot day, it is best to eat only a salad. Salads are wet and cooling.

Eating according to the season is very important. In winter, eat soups, root vegetables and warming foods. Nature provides the right season and location of foods; man tries to tamper with Nature by picking food before it is ripe, shipping it long distances, growing it unnaturally in hot houses with artificial chemical fertilizers. So, eat according to the seasons. If you enjoy tropical fruits, move to the tropics (if you can). Even tropical fruits have their seasons. In order for these fruits to be shipped to northern countries, they are picked green and sprayed to preserve them. They are not the true fruit.

Eat a wide variety of foods. Stay away from excesses —over-eating, over-salting and over-use of sugar (no sugar and no salt are best of all). Also, to avoid food allergies eat from a wide variety of food groups. Eating the same foods every day stresses the immune system, because the foods become allergenic. Wheat, milk, corn, soy, yeast, chocolate, tea, coffee, beef, citrus, shellfish, eggs and potatoes are common allergenic foods. No foods are free from causing allergenic reactions, but these are the most common. Rather than being a nourishing substance, the food turns into a toxin or poison.

Often, when a person is admitted to a hospital suffering from pneumonia, the first thing he is fed is chicken. Because the body temperature of chicken is higher, it raises the body temperature of the patient about seven percent. Consequently, many people die of excessive fever.

Foods that are good for the AIDS patient are carrots and grapes. Both must be free from pesticides. We are not writing ''organic'' because ''organic'' does not necessarily mean that no pesticides were used; it means that the conditions in which they were grown were natural—e.g., no chemical fertilizers were used in the growing. Certain fruits and vegetables could be grown without being sprayed but later their surfaces are treated with toxic substances for preservation and shipping. These substances can be wax, biphenyl, etc. (See below.)

Grapes contain cell salts which nourish the blood system. Carrots—raw or juiced preferably (cooked, second choice)—are beneficial for AIDS patients because of the nutrients they contain—especially Beta-Carotene. Other good foods with this valuable substance are: beets and beet juice; citrus fruits; yellow and orange squashes, sweet potatoes and yams.

STRESS IN FOOD ANIMALS

It has been found that rates of immune dysfunction in animals can be varied tremendously by the stress under which the animals are placed. Highly stressed animals have immune system dysfunctions and a much greater incidence of cancer than comparable animals housed in low-stress conditions.

Psychological and physical causes could be: overcrowding;

drugs; lack of exercise, fresh air or sunshine; separation (such as the calf being taken from the cow); constant milking; and all other forms of abuse toward the food animals in our society. The fear and terror that the animals who are about to be killed feel—the seeing and hearing and smelling of death—being consciously aware of what is happening to their fellows ahead of them—all this results in tremendous stress, the production of toxins, and disease. THIS IS PASSED ON TO THE HUMANS CONSUMING THEIR FLESH!

Dr. Virginia Livingston-Wheeler has been a cancer researcher for 40 years. She discovered that the majority of chickens are infected with cancer. Very few of the cancerous growths are cut out during the factory processing, because of the speed of the assembly line. Even when a section IS cut out, the pathogen is in the bloodstream, hence throughout the body of the chicken. What we have today is:

SICK FOOD ANIMALS = SICK MEAT = SICK PEOPLE

DO YOU KNOW WHAT YOU ARE EATING TODAY?

(by Dr. Philip J. Welsh, D.D.S., N.D.—with permission)

ABOUT ORANGES: All unripe citrus fruits harm the tooth enamel and the intestinal tract lining, so watch the oranges you buy and eat.

It is customary now for the big citrus growers to treat (embalm) their fruits with a biphenyl compound. My first experience with this problem occurred a number of years ago before I ever knew about this process of treating fruits.

My wife and I had eaten some oranges from the supermarket. Shortly afterwards, we both began to itch, mostly on the chest and nose. It did not take me long to conclude that the oranges had been treated, because this was the only food we both had eaten. I returned to the supermarket and asked the produce man to show me the box in which these oranges were packed. Upon close examination, I finally found a sentence, in very small print, which stated: "This fruit has been treated with biphenyl to preserve its freshness." I asked the produce man about this. He had never heard of the process nor knew anything about it.

Then I talked with the girl at the fresh juice bar in the supermarket. She was squeezing these same oranges. I asked her whether she knew anything about this chemical. She told me she did not. However, she added that she had to wear rubber gloves to protect her hands when cutting and handling the oranges. If she did not wear the gloves, her hands would swell and itch. I then informed her about the printing on the box.

Biphenyl is a chemical which is used to embalm living matter, and is extremely harmful to the human body.

This shows how important it is not to use orange peel or lemon peel in your recipes, unless the fruit is organically grown.

PREPARE YOURSELF FOR A SHOCK!

To Maintain
FRESHNESS

IN TRANSIT—THIS FRUIT HAS BEEN

PROTECTED WITH BIPHENYL,
2,4-DICHLOROPHENOXYACETATE
AND SODIUM O-PHENYLPHENATE

While writing this section for this edition, we got the idea of tracking down more information on the chemical biphenyl.

If they use it to embalm our fruits, could it possibly be the same chemical that is used to embalm corpses in preparation for a good appearance in the casket at the funeral?

We telephoned a local mortuary, which confirmed that this was so. We were given the number of the chemical company, which further confirmed it. "YES, IT IS BIPHENYL THAT IS USED EXTENSIVELY IN THE EMBALMING PROCESS IN MORTUARIES!"

It is unbelievable what they are doing to the food today. *You should do everything you can to protect yourself.* Also, do whatever you can to stop such practices, or join organizations that are working against food adulteration.

Is it any wonder that millions of Americans have cancer, arthritis, and other degenerative diseases?

Now Look at This:

The following menu is translated into the *preservatives and additives* likely to be contained in the very foods you may be eating today. Here is what you could be eating for LUNCH or DINNER:

JUICE:
Benzoic acid (preservative)
Dimethyl polysiloxane (anti-foaming agent)

FRUIT CUP:
Calcium hypochlorite (germicide wash)
Sodium chloride (prevents browning)
Sodium hydroxide (peeling agent)

Calcium hydroxide (firming agent)
Sodium metasilicate (peeling agent—peaches)
Sorbic acid (fungistat)
Sulfur dioxide (preservative)
FD & C Red No. 3 (coloring for cherries)

SOUP:
Butylated hydroxyanisole (anti-oxidant)
Dimethyl polysiloxane (anti-foaming agent)
Sodium phosphate dibasic (emulsion for tomato soup)
Citric acid (dispersant in soup base)

SANDWICH: MEAT & PROCESSED CHEESE
Sodium diacetate (mold inhibitor)
Mono-glyceride (emulsifier)
Potassium bromate (maturing agent)
Aluminum phosphate (improver)
Calcium phosphate monobasic (dough conditioner)
Aluminum potassium sulfate (acid-baking powder
    ingredient)
Ascorbate (anti-oxidant)
Sodium or potassium nitrate (color fixative)
Sodium chloride (preservative)
Guar gum (binder)
Hydrogen peroxide (bleach and bactericide)
Nordihydroguariaretic acid (anti-oxidant)
Alkanate (dye)
Methylviolet (marking ink)
Asafoetide (onion flavoring)
Sodium phosphate (buffer)
Magnesium carbonate (drying agent)
Calcium propionate (preservative)
Calcium citrate (plasticizer)
Sodium citrate (emulsifier)
Sodium alginate (stabilizer)

Acetic acid (acid)
Phroligneous acid (smoke flavor)
Chloramine T (flour bleach)
Chloramine T (deodorant)

FRUIT PIE:
Sodium diacetate (mold inhibitor)
Sorbic acid (fungistat)
Butylated hydroxyanisole (anti-oxidant)
Sodium sulfite (anti-browning)
Mono- and di-glycerides (emulsifiers)
Aluminum ammonium sulfate (acid)
FD & C Red No. 3 (cherry coloring)
Calcium chloride (apple pie mix firming agent)
Potassium bromate (maturing agent)
Calcium carbonate (neutralizer)

COMMERCIAL ICE CREAM:
Diethyl glycol (used instead of eggs, it is an anti-freeze
    and paint remover)
Piperonal (used in place of vanilla, it is a lice killer)
Ethyl acetate (used in place of pineapple, it is a cleaner
    for leather and textiles)
Butyraldehyde (used instead of nuts, it is one of the
    ingredients of rubber cement)
Amyl acetate (used for banana flavor; an oil paint
    solvent)
Benzyl acetate (used for strawberry flavor; a solvent)

Do you know that you can make a delicious and healthful ice milk by using any of the following ingredients:
milk, honey, fresh fruit, pure vanilla and carob powder for
a chocolate-type flavoring?

After reading about the many chemical additives that are
put into our foods, one can see why so many people are

suffering with many diseases. Over 3,000 additives are used in the manufacture of the food we eat. Some estimates of individual consumption are as high as five pounds a year! Even experts cannot agree on the safety of or necessity for all these chemicals.

The deadliest enemies of nations are not their foreign foes; they always dwell within their own borders.
>   —WILLIAM JAMES, 1911

The use of drugs in the U.S. today is one of these foes that could destroy our nation; crime is another, and every citizen can think of other foes within, out of control.

Oh, that the medical doctors of the world—so respected —so heavily trained—and to whom the vast majority of the public looks for guidance in matters of health, life and death—would make a turn-around in their methods—and learn to teach the people nutrition and other preventive methods, and alternative, natural therapies. But first, the medical schools must change their curricula; doctors must be taught differently.

A polluted body, full of toxins, cannot be cured by adding more poisons (drugs)—but only by purifying the body in every possible way—as outlined in this book.

Thomas A. Edison, many years ago, made this prophecy: "The doctor of the future will give no medicine, but will interest his patients in the care of the human frame, in diet, in the cause and prevention of disease."

—

SEVEN

—

PROGRESSIVE AND SEQUENTIAL EATING; MENUS AND RECIPES

A natural, body-building diet consists of nutritiously simple and easily digested foods. Heavy, rich sauces, meats, and foods poorly combined not only hinder absorption, but putrify and clog the digestive tract. For maximum absorption, eat fruits by themselves, non-starchy vegetables with protein foods, low starchy vegetables and carbohydrates together, and all melons by themselves.

When proteins are combined properly, they complement each other; they increase the quality and quantity of the protein available for your body to use.

Protein is one of the more difficult food factors to digest. Each type of protein requires different timing and different digestive secretions. Each different type of protein should be eaten at different meals. For example: eggs, fish, cheese, nuts should be eaten at different meals.

Acid and protein combinations are poor because the acid interferes with the gastric flow. It is acceptable to eat acid fruits with protein foods, such as nuts, seeds or cheese, because the fruit acids do not interfere with the flow of gastric juices, due to the high fat content.

For maximum absorption of fat-soluble vitamins (A, D, E and K), a small quantity of cold-pressed, unrefined vegetable oil is used; it increases the absorption of these nutrients.

The three big vitamins that have proven to be most deficient in degenerative disease are: niacin, thiamine, and pantothenic acid. The required quantities of these vitamins

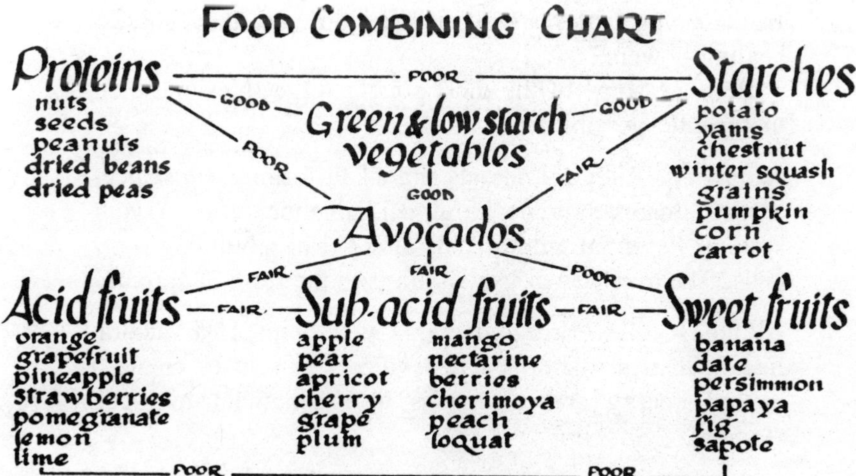

cannot always be available in our foods, so supplementation of all the B vitamins is highly recommended.

Proper food combining suggests that most proteins have sufficient fat content, and it is not necessary to add more. This means flesh foods do not need extra butter, or nuts, or avocado, or oils.

Sugars and starches are a poor food combination. A whole-grain cereal and orange juice is an example of poor food combining; the sugar in the orange juice delays the starch digestion, so bacterial fermentation takes place. The salivary secretion does not contain amylase (an enzyme that digests starch); therefore, the sugars are delayed in the stomach.

THE HEALING POWERS OF VEGETABLES

Because vegetables are so rich in nutrients, they possess healing powers.

Here are some of the most popular vegetables and their therapeutic possibilities:

ALFALFA: Rich in minerals and alkali-forming substances to help maintain a healthful acid-alkaline ratio in your system. Essential amino acids also aid in rebuilding body cells. The best way to use alfalfa is in the form of sprouts.

ARTICHOKE: Prime mineral source with 15% natural insulin that is hydrolized to levulose by acid to create a natural energy source that is also beneficial to weak stomachs.

ASPARAGUS: Abundant in vitamins and minerals, especially Vitamin A which is needed for visual sharpness.

BEET: High mineral content aids in bloodstream nourishment and activated lymphatic flow throughout the circulatory system.

BROCCOLI: High in vitamins and minerals to maintain adequate water balance of your body.

CABBAGE: Successfully used by Dr. Cheney (through freshly squeezed raw juice) as a means of treating stomach ulcers, both peptic and duodenal. Dr. Ann Wigmore of the Hippocrates Health Institute, Boston, also uses raw cabbage juice and raw cabbage for healing.

CELERY: Excellent vitamin source and aids in nervous disorders by helping to rid the body of carbon dioxide, a toxic waste product.

ENDIVE: Nature's own laxative, helps in conditions of indigestion and liver ailments because of its rich Vitamin A and C content.

KALE: A top-notch source of Vitamins A and C, needed for better vision, skin and hair health.

LETTUCE: Rich in nerve-strengthening minerals and aids in conditions of excess stomach acidity and constipation. Also good source of chlorophyll.

MUSHROOMS: Good B-complex source, as well as B_{12} needed for blood enrichment.

MUSTARD GREENS: Tangy taste, high in capillary-building Vitamin C.

OKRA: Valuable because it has such a low carbohydrate content which is beneficial for those on reducing diets. Also rich in iron and calcium and aids in conditions of colitis, intestinal disorders.

ONION: While not very popular because of its pungent

odor, it is rich in minerals and vitamins and stimulates the gastric tract. A slice of raw onion in a vegetable salad is a popular method of serving.

PEAS: All varieties of peas have much protein and minerals.

PEPPER: Juice is rich in silicon to nourish your hair, skin and nails; good for those who are troubled by skin blemishes.

RADISHES: High in magnesium to soothe your nerves and stimulate a natural digestive flow. High sulfur content cleanses your bloodstream and aids in its purification.

TOMATO: The best source available of B_2 and C, plus vegetable amino acids. Highly alkaline because of its superior mineral content, the tomato helps to neutralize excessively acid stomach conditions caused by over-eating of starchy foods.

THE BEST WAYS TO PREPARE: These are best raw: alfalfa, celery, endive, lettuce, radishes, tomato.

Other vegetables: steam lightly. Artichokes need to be cooked. Beets can be grated or juiced.

The worst ways to prepare are: frying, or in mixtures such as casseroles.

The AIDS patient should stay with our recommendations in this book. Not all of the vegetables in this list are recommended for AIDS patients. Mushrooms should be eliminated if there is a Candida Albicans problem.

THE TEMPERATURES OF FOODS

Foods should be neither too hot nor too cold. Especially when the person is sick, this is important, in order not to burden the digestive process. Food should be at room temperature. Too often people take food right out of the refrigerator and eat it.

Cold drinks with ice are a shock to the digestive organs. They cause the stomach to contract; digestion cannot occur, and stones can form over a period of time—especially if one eats fat and simultaneously drinks iced liquids. The fats harden and block passage in the digestive tract, and lodge where they are deposited. This can cause tumors, and is a possible cause of cysts and arteriosclerosis. A simple experiment that can be done in your kitchen is to take a greasy plate with animal fat on it, and place it under cold water. The fat will congeal. Eggs are also notorious for doing this.

In Oriental medicine diagnosis, a damp spleen condition (excessive wetness in the "lower burner") is due to excessive amounts of wet, raw, cold food.

Salads should be eaten at room temperature, preferably in the sunshine.

Here is an experience from our own lives. We, the authors, visited a raw food restaurant in Los Angeles, and dined. The salad bar had much ice underneath the bowls of salads, and the dressings were likewise iced.

During and after our meal, we both shivered and felt unwell, although the temperature was the usual warmth of Southern California in the summertime.

(We understand the problems of restaurants—they must keep the salads from spoiling. Hence the conclusion that we can eat better food at home than at restaurants.)

Contrariwise, very hot liquids, such as coffee and tea, are also very harmful. And drinking very hot coffee several times a day is a national habit, unfortunately. Excessively hot drinks are physical irritants to the mucous membranes.

These physical irritants can cause all kinds of health

problems, including cancer—and can contribute to AIDS.

Have you ever noticed how much better food tastes when eaten out of doors? Consider what would be the ideal setting for a meal. It would be by a lake, stream or ocean, or in the mountains, in a forest, near trees, with sunshine warming us and our foods, in a relaxed frame of mind. Beautiful, harmonious music would be a plus. This would be an ideal setting. Such a place is called Eden, Elysium, or Paradise. We should try to approximate this as much as possible in our lives. People who live in the country can do so—and more people should leave the cities—to get back to Nature—for better health, more normal lives, more peace and happiness in their lives—and a healthy longevity.

PROGRESSIVE HEALTHFUL MENUS FOR THE AIDS PATIENT

Whatever the season, Nature naturally provides the cure.

Upon rising, do the routine described in Chapter 5, "Natural Treatment," before eating anything. The body is most toxic before going to sleep and upon rising, due to the lactic acid build-up. Eat the first meal at 11:00 A.M., approximately.

Because the digestive forces are in a weakened state, proper food combining must be utilized. As the digestive forces are made stronger, more kinds of food can be tolerated. Be sure not to use salt or sugar.

THIS IS COOKING FOR THE SICK. The food is simple, easily digested, and does not contain any denatured, refined carbohydrates, such as white flour or sugar. No rancid oils or stale foods are used. The freshest food obtainable should be found, prepared, and eaten. YOUR BODY DESERVES IT!

THE FIRST FIVE DAYS: Consecutive eating. This means starting with the easiest to digest, liquid foods, and simple foods, and progressing to more complex foods.

MENUS AND RECIPES

THE FIRST DAY

11:00 A.M.—Drink 8 ounces of pure, freshly pressed carrot juice, from peeled carrots, or a carrot-celery combination.
- Blended Salad (see recipe, page 106) with Romaine or Butter lettuce, cucumber (peeled if not organic), vine-ripened tomatoes, lemon juice, olive oil (extra virgin —cold pressed).
- Raw Salad—anise root, lettuce, steamed beets and cucumbers.
- Two lightly cooked fertile egg yolks.
- Supplementation taken with food.

2:00 P.M.—SECOND MEAL—drink pure, freshly made carrot juice, as before.
- Blended salad.
- Raw salad with unsalted olives.
- Freshly roasted, unsalted seeds—pumpkin or sunflower.

DINNER—6:00–7:00 P.M.
- Take digestive enzyme.
- Puree of fresh asparagus (very good for cleaning the system).
- Two baked potatoes. "Yellow Finns" are organic —an excellent potato, extremely alkaline, and very tasty. Eat the peels, too. Eat with cold-pressed olive oil and red beet powder sprinkled on top. (These are digestive aids.)

- Steamed green beans (organic if possible; help maintain proper blood sugar levels).

9:00 P.M.
- Fresh blueberries (if in season) sprinkled with Perrier Cartier green clay. Eat the blueberries and drink the clay water. Tastes good and deposits minerals into the system. Blueberries are good for the glandular system.
- If not available, have an organic baked apple with rice syrup or barley malt syrup, or raisins, for sweetness.

> Most of these meals are quickly prepared. They are all nutritious. The less complicated the combinations, the better absorption.

BLENDED SALAD—*7 minutes*

Why blended salads? In sequential eating, you go from simple to complex. Blended salads take the burden off the digestive system and prepare it for more complex digestion. These recipes are all planned for one person.

Butter lettuce, 1 head, OR
Romaine lettuce, ½ head
Cucumber, ½ (unpeeled if organic)
Lemon juice, 1 teaspoon
Tomato, 1, vine-ripened
Olive oil (cold pressed, extra virgin), 2 teaspoons

The lettuce should be washed and dried. It may be rinsed in tap water with 1 tablespoon chlorine bleach or a mild natural cleaner, and then rinsed thoroughly in pure water. Dry with a paper or cloth towel. This procedure is important when the lettuce is not organic; it will reduce the toxic sprays and also kill larvae and bugs on the lettuce.

Put all the ingredients into the blender, and blend briefly, until the mixture is a puree. Serve in bowl with spoon. Even though it is blended, the person should salivate it before swallowing, for best assimilation.

(This food and most of our recipes here are also good for infants and the elderly, and all sick persons.)

RAW SALAD—*10 minutes*

(All vegetables organic, if possible.)

> Lettuce (Butter, 1 head) or Romaine (½ head)
> Green bell pepper (1, washed)
> Anise root (½)
> Celery (not bleached, as is found in the supermarkets) (1 stalk)
> Tomato, 1, vine-ripened
> Lemon juice, 2 tablespoons
> Olive oil (cold pressed, extra virgin), 2 teaspoons

Lettuce is best torn with the fingers, before serving; it oxidizes less. Chop the other vegetables finely, just before serving. (Vegetables oxidate quickly once they are cut.) Use different cuts for eye appeal.

SALADS SHOULD HAVE ONE ROOT VEGETABLE (carrots, finely grated, turnips, jicama), ONE VEGETA-BLE THAT GROWS ABOVE THE GROUND (green pepper, cucumber, tomato), and ONE LEAFY VEGETA-BLE. Any kind of lettuce may be used except Iceberg lettuce, which is bleached. Belgian endive is good.

SOFT SIMMERED EGGS—*7 minutes*

Eggs, 2, fertile if possible

An egg should never be boiled. Put the eggs in a pan of boiling water. Let them simmer without a flame or other heat. Eat the yolk only.

More hydrochloric acid is present in the stomach at the beginning of the meal, so we recommend eating the egg yolk first, before the salad.

FRESH SEEDS—*5 minutes*

Husked sunflower and pumpkin seeds can be slightly dry roasted until they pop, in a skillet. These seeds can be sprinkled on the tops of salads or be eaten with fruits.

PUREE OF FRESH ASPARAGUS—*10 minutes*

Fresh asparagus, ½ to 1 pound
Olive oil, ½ teaspoon

Cut off the white, tough portion. Wash, cut the asparagus in half. Put the fibrous portion on the bottom of the steamer, the flower portion on top. Use filtered or distilled water when steaming vegetables. The reason is: the pollutants and chemicals in the water do pollute the food, so try to use the best water possible.

Steam until tender, cool, put into a blender, add the olive oil, and serve.

BAKED POTATOES—*45 minutes/1 hour*

2 medium-sized potatoes (Idaho or Yellow Finn preferred)
Red beet powder
Olive oil (cold pressed, extra virgin)
Nori

Thoroughly wash and scrub the potatoes. Set the oven temperature to 450° and on "bake." Put potatoes on rack in oven when it is hot and bake until done. Test for doneness. The potatoes should be crispy on the outside and soft on the inside. Split in half and sprinkle on red beet powder (from a natural food store). Red beet powder contains betaine hydrochloride, which aids digestion. Add the olive oil, and Nori instead of salt. Nori is seaweed, which comes in sheets or flakes. If you use sheets, roast before using.

STEAMED GREEN BEANS—*5–6 minutes*

Green beans (quantity desired)
Pure water

Leave the beans whole, and steam. Green beans are extremely alkaline, and greatly benefit hypoglycemia (low blood sugar) because of the chromium content.

FRESH BLUEBERRIES WITH GREEN CLAY

Wash berries in spring water, sprinkle with green clay (from a natural food store); place in refrigerator. Eat when cool.

ORGANIC BAKED APPLE—*30 minutes*

1 or 2 medium-sized apples
  (baking apple such as Rome Beauty)
2 teaspoons ground almonds
2 teaspoons raisins
Barley malt or rice syrup for sweetness (2 teaspoons per
  apple)

Remove core, place almonds and raisins in the center, pour barley malt or rice syrup over the tops of the apples.

Place in 350° oven and bake for 30 minutes.

THE SECOND DAY

11:00 A.M.—Drink a warm, herbal tea of your choice.
* Eat "Bianca's Compote"—a combination of organic, dried fruits (prunes, figs, raisins, etc.)
* Supplementation.

2:00 P.M.—SECOND MEAL—drink pure, freshly made carrot juice, as before.
* Blended salad
* Raw salad
* 6 ounces of well-cooked, short-grain, brown rice (called *ojia* by the Japanese), on the wet side.
* Supplementation.
DINNER—6:00–7:00 P.M.
* Garlic-caraway seed consommé
* Steamed cabbage or Brussels sprouts or broccoli or cauliflower, with lemon-tahini sauce.
* One baked seasonal squash.
* 8 ounces of cooked beans: either mung, lentil, white Northern, chickpea, azuki. (Pinto beans have too much oil, for this sequential period.)
* Fruit Kanten Custard for dessert.

BIANCA'S COMPOTE—*5 minutes*

(Use dried, unsulfured fruits. Use any or all of these.)

Greek Calmyra figs
Sun-ripened raisins

Black Mission figs
Prunes
Pure water
Lemon, ½

Place the fruit in a large jar; add hot water and the lemon. The lemon allows the iron in the fruit to be leached into the juice. Let stand 24 hours, either in the refrigerator or outside of it. This makes an ideal food which can start the day, but use sparingly. It is sweet; use in moderation.

RICE CREAM OR RICE *OJIA* [Japanese]—*45 minutes*

1 cup rice—organic, short-grained, brown
2½–3 cups pure water

Roast the rice lightly in a skillet, then place in the water. Bring to a boil, turn down and simmer. Keep adding water. It becomes a type of rice soup—well cooked, very nutritious, easily digested, and is loaded with B vitamins.

CARAWAY SEED SOUP—*15 minutes*

½ onion
⅛ cup pure water, plus 1 more cup
1 clove garlic
½ stalk celery, chopped
1 teaspoon caraway seeds
½ teaspoon olive oil
Croutons from toasted wheat bread

Put the olive oil into a pan, add the onion, chopped, and sauté lightly. Add the ⅛ cup water, and on a low flame, let the mixture simmer for 10 minutes. Add the clove of garlic, finely minced, the chopped celery (add a few of the leaves), sprinkle the caraway seeds into it, and add the 1 cup of pure water.

This makes 1 cup of soup. Toast whole-wheat bread, cut into cubes, to make croutons, and sprinkle on top.

STEAMED BROCCOLI, BRUSSELS SPROUTS or CAULIFLOWER—*12 to 15 minutes*

Cut or break the broccoli or cauliflower apart; rinse the Brussels sprouts well. Place these in a steamer which sits in a large pan. There should be enough water in the bottom of the pan to reach the steamer. Steam until a bright color appears in the vegetables; they are done. Immediately add the sauce (see below), and serve.

LEMON-TAHINI SAUCE FOR VEGETABLES
—*10 minutes*

2 tablespoons natural tahini or sesame seed butter
½ clove garlic, minced
¼ lemon, squeezed
Dash or $\frac{1}{16}$ teaspoon kelp powder
Pure water

Take the tahini or sesame seed butter, the minced garlic, 2 TB of water, the lemon juice and the kelp powder. Bring this to a boil, turn down the heat and simmer; add a little more water to make a creamy consistency and pour, warm, over steamed vegetables.

COOKED BEANS—*1½ hours*

(Use mung, azuki, white Northern, garbanzo beans, chick peas or lentils.)

1 cup beans
2 cups pure water
Pinch of fresh ginger
⅛ clove garlic
¼ green pepper
¼ onion

Soak the beans overnight. Drain off the water. To cook, put 12 ounces of water, just to cover the beans 2 inches over the top. Use 1 cup beans. Boil; pour off all the liquid. Add fresh water. Bring to a boil again, down to a simmer, cook for 1 hour 15 minutes, adding water when needed. For flavor, you may add fresh ginger, garlic, green pepper, or onion (one or all).

FRUIT KANTEN CUSTARD—*½ hour*

1 stick or flake of agar-agar
1 quart natural fruit juice, unsweetened
1 cup fresh, sweet fruit
   (non-citrus; apples are good)
2 tablespoons sesame tahini

This dessert is made from agar-agar, which is a non-caloric, non-animal-derived gelatin, from algae. It has body-building nutrients in it. It comes in sticks or flakes. Buy in the Japanese section of a supermarket. Be sure it does not have any artificial coloring in it.

Take the natural fruit juice, pour into a large pot; add the agar-agar, 1 stick per quart. Bring to a boil, turn down the heat and cover. Fresh fruit can be cut in small pieces and cooked in this liquid, on a small simmer, for 10 minutes. It is then turned off and the sesame tahini is folded into the mixture. It is then poured in fruit cups and refrigerated.

THE THIRD DAY

11:00 A.M.—Fresh grapefruit (very high in magnesium and hesperidin) with organic walnuts.
* Buckwheat groats with garlic (high in rutin and hesperidin).
* Supplementation.

1:00 P.M.—Raw, organic Concord grapes, if in season. Or fresh cherries.

2:00 P.M.—SECOND MEAL—Drink freshly made carrot juice, as before (organic, peeled carrots)
* Blended salad.
* Raw salad made from local, organic, non-bitter vegetables: Romaine; green pepper (unwaxed); sunflower seed sprouts; buckwheat lettuce sprouts. (You can sprout your own.) The dressing is lemon or lime juice combined with olive oil.

DINNER—6:00–7:00 P.M.
* Digestive enzymes.
* Raw, unheated, home-made cottage cheese, from high-quality unpasteurized, unsalted milk. Tempeh burger with root vegetable stew, containing: daikon white radish, burdock root, taro, wild Japanese yam *(Toro ro imo* or *jinengo)*. This has lots of vitamins and minerals.

9:00 P.M.—A fresh apple or pear may be eaten. (As always, try to find organic fruit.)

It is best if vegetables are served at room temperature. Even better, place raw vegetables in the sunshine before eating.

BUCKWHEAT GROATS or KASHA—*20 minutes*

1 stalk scallions
1 clove garlic
1 cup unroasted buckwheat
2 cups water
1 teaspoon sunflower or pumpkin seeds

Buy buckwheat raw, because the roasted is overdone. Place the raw buckwheat in a skillet and lightly roast it, about 5 minutes. At the same time, boil the pure water. While the buckwheat is still hot from being pan roasted, pour boiling water over it, and turn down to a simmer, and let the buckwheat absorb the water and simmer for about 20 minutes.

You may add the other items, for more flavor.

THE FOURTH DAY

11:00 A.M.—Drink pure, warm water with fresh lemon juice. It has lots of calcium and vitamin C, and helps the liver.

FAST FROM FOOD UNTIL YOUR LUNCH.

2:00 P.M.
- A bowl of vegetable-barley soup. Brown rice cake spread with fresh nut butter.
- Supplementation.
- Raw salad.

DINNER—6:00–7:00 P.M.
- Supplementation.
- Two egg yolks (from soft-boiled eggs).
- Two steamed vegetables—beets, peas.
Two hours later—Dessert: frozen banana, mixed with another fruit; put it through a blender.

VEGETABLE-BARLEY SOUP—*35 minutes*

Select vegetables of your choice:
  2 stalks celery
  1 carrot
  1 teaspoon dehydrated mushrooms (preferably Shiitake)
  1 fresh tomato
  ¼ head cabbage
  2½–3 cups pure water
  1 teaspoon vegetable seasoning (in place of salt)
  1 sheet kombu (seaweed)

This is an excellent meal for the sick. Sauté the dehydrated vegetables in water (this eliminates oil) for 5 minutes; add the carrots and celery, and water sauté them until tender.

Wipe the kombu sheet; soak for 10 minutes. Take the liquid from it (dashi—the soaking juice), and pour into the soup pan. Add the washed barley. Add water, bring to a boil; turn down and simmer. If it gets too thick while cooking, add water. Add the vegetable seasoning.

We have said that the cooking time is 35–40 minutes; actually, you need to cook until the barley is soft.

HERE ARE FOOD ITEMS THAT STIMULATE HORMONE PRODUCTION. They can be added to recipes.

CAYENNE PEPPER, taken in small doses (5–7 grains), will help boost a sluggish system. The pepper may be combined with hot or cold water. It is a very high source of Vitamin A. But large quantities of cayenne irritate the mucous membrane of the digestive system.

CUCUMBERS also stimulate hormone production because of the Vitamin E content. They should be organic; if they are not, be sure to peel them.

THE FIFTH DAY

11:00 A.M.—An herbal tea of your choice.
* Millet (a cooked cereal) with oat cream sauce.

2:00 P.M.—SECOND MEAL
* Blended salad.
* Raw salad.
* 6 ounces of raw, unsalted, unprocessed Monterey Jack cheese. (This cheese is not highly fermented; many AIDS patients have Candida Albicans; fermented foods feed this fungus.)
* Supplementation. As absorption is increased by now, supplementation is increased.

DINNER—6:00–7:00 P.M.
* A small quantity of steamed, mild, white fish, with fresh lemon.
* Steamed kale.
* Baked yam.

MILLET WITH OAT CREAM—*45 minutes*

1 cup millet
½ cup organic raw oats
2½ cups pure water

First rinse the millet thoroughly; then dry (pan) roast. This grain lends itself to pressure cooking, because when boiled, it often becomes too mushy. Pressure-cook for 30 minutes or cook for 45 minutes in regular pot.

Serve warm with oatmeal cream sauce. Take the raw oats and make an oatmeal with water to pour over the top. This aids the digestion of the millet, makes it more moist.

STEAMED KALE—*12–15 minutes*

The kale should be washed and chopped. It must not be over-cooked, but be soft and palatable. Steam no more than 6 minutes, and eat immediately before it turns color.

BAKED YAM—*35–40 minutes*

1 large or 2 small yams.
(Try to buy them in a natural food store; those found in supermarkets are usually heavily sprayed.)

Bake yams in the skin, at 350 degrees.

THE SIXTH DAY

11:00 A.M.—Freshly prepared carrot juice, as before.
- Steel-cut oats, sprinkled with freshly roasted seeds (pumpkin seeds have high amounts of zinc) and cinnamon.
- Supplementation.

2:00 P.M.—SECOND MEAL
- Vegetarian tostada.
- Steamed collard greens with sweet, unsalted, raw butter.
- Avocado, lettuce, grated carrots and beets, on a bed of a bean tortilla; tahini sauce.
- Supplementation.

4:00 P.M.—Banana-rice custard.

DINNER: None (patient fasts this evening).

TOSTADA SUPREME—*10 minutes*

1 slice organic, round, flat, unsalted whole-wheat bread
⅛ cup cooked kidney beans
2 leaves lettuce
¼ cup each grated carrots and grated beets
Gazpacho or lemon-tahini dressing or natural salsa

Bake the bread in oven until crisp. Spread the beans on the bottom, add the lettuce and grated beets and carrots. Add one of the sauces, which can be purchased.

BANANA-RICE CUSTARD—*10 minutes*

2 or more cups cooked, brown rice
   (several days old gives it more flavor)
1 cup organic apple juice
Pinch of cinnamon (optional)
2 bananas, ripe
Vanilla, ⅛ teaspoon
1 tablespoon sesame tahini
Fresh mint for garnish (optional)

Pour apple juice over the rice, let it stand, preferably overnight. Put the rice, apple juice, banana, vanilla and other ingredients into a blender. Blend lightly. Add fresh mint as a garnish, if available. If it is too thick, you may add more apple juice; if too thin, add more rice. The consistency should be creamy as a custard.

THE SEVENTH DAY

11:00 A.M.—Carrot juice, with daikon juice (expels mucus)
   —freshly pressed.
• Supplementation.

2:00 P.M.—SECOND MEAL
* Blended salad
* Whole grain noodles with tomato sauce. (Both should have no salt or preservatives. You can find these in the health food section of your supermarket or a health food store.) Noodles derived from Jerusalem artichokes are especially good for individuals who have wheat allergies. A small amount of fresh, unsalted raw butter can be placed on the noodles.

DINNER—6:00–7:00 P.M.
* Supplementation.
* Large, raw salad with scallions, almonds, butter lettuce, avocado.
* Steamed, fresh sweet corn (if in season). Use fresh, raw, unsalted butter.
* If not available, use Yellow Finn potatoes, baked, or Hubbard squash, baked.
* Cucumber, grated carrots.
* Whole grain bread (unsalted. yeast-free).

JINENJO NOODLES—*30 minutes*

1 package jinenjo noodles
2 or 3 tomatoes
⅛ teaspoon oregano, fresh if possible
⅛ teaspoon thyme, fresh if possible
1 tablespoon olive oil (extra virgin, cold pressed)
½ clove garlic
⅛ teaspoon dehydrated onion

Make a tomato sauce with the fresh tomatoes in the blender, with the oregano and thyme. At the same time, boil water and add the noodles; cook until soft but firm. Combine the other ingredients with the tomato sauce; add the sauce on top of the noodles, and serve.

HOME-MADE COTTAGE CHEESE—*4 hours*

1 quart buttermilk
Juice from ½ lemon

Use a large glass or earthenware bowl. Add the lemon juice to the buttermilk, and stir. Place the mixture in the oven under very low heat, about 120 degrees. In 4 or 5 hours the buttermilk will form a thick clabber and separate from the whey. Pour the entire mixture into a cheesecloth bag, hang the bag over a bowl, and allow the whey to drain into the bowl. The remainder in the cheesecloth bag is a fine, delicious, delicate cheese, better than any you can buy. Place in a glass jar and store in the refrigerator. Do not discard the whey. It can be used as a nourishing and rejuvenating drink. Note that the higher the temperature the harder the cheese.

May we warn you against store-bought cottage cheese? It has much salt, and (believe it or not) also plaster of Paris (to hold it together).

TEMPEH BURGER—*10 minutes*

Unsalted tempeh patty (a soybean product)
Olive oil

These can be purchased in natural food stores. Be sure they are unsalted. Bake in oven with a little fresh olive oil on top. Do not fry.

You may season the burger with Vegenaise (a non-dairy mayonnaise made with lecithin), or a natural mustard without vinegar or salt.

ROOT VEGETABLE STEW—*1 hour*

(Asian or natural food stores have the ingredients)

   3 strips kombu seaweed
   2 medium roots daikon (white radish)
   2 medium roots burdock
   3 taro roots
   Wild mountain potato (*jinenjo* or *toro ro imo)*
      (about 6 inches)
   2 carrots
   1 yam
   Onions
   Konnyaku: wild Japanese plant (½ package, sliced thin)

Wipe the kombu seaweed with a cloth; soak for 20 minutes in about 3 cups of water; they swell. Separate the kombu from the liquid, which is called dashi. Put the dashi into the container to be used. Wash and peel the daikon. Wash but do not peel the burdock root (cut off the ends). The taro root and wild mountain potato are washed and peeled. The pieces should be cut large and circular.

The konnyaku is derived from a herb and has a rubbery gelatin consistency; it is very nutritious.

Add the carrots, chopped in big pieces. Onions can be added for flavor, and you may add a yam for sweetness. Lightly "water sauté" these vegetables in a skillet until they brown. Cover them with the dashi and put the pieces of kombu over the top. Put a lid on it and cook for about 1 hour.

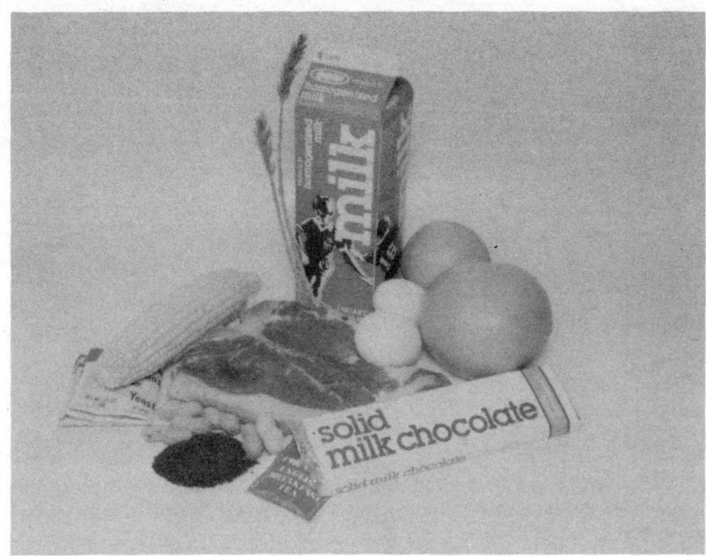

P-1

ALLERGIES. The most common allergenic foods are: wheat, milk, corn, soy, yeast, chocolate, tea, coffee, beef, citrus, shellfish, eggs, potatoes and peanuts. Allergies are a partial cause of Candida Albicans, and are also deleterious to the immune system because the body has to work harder to get rid of the toxins.

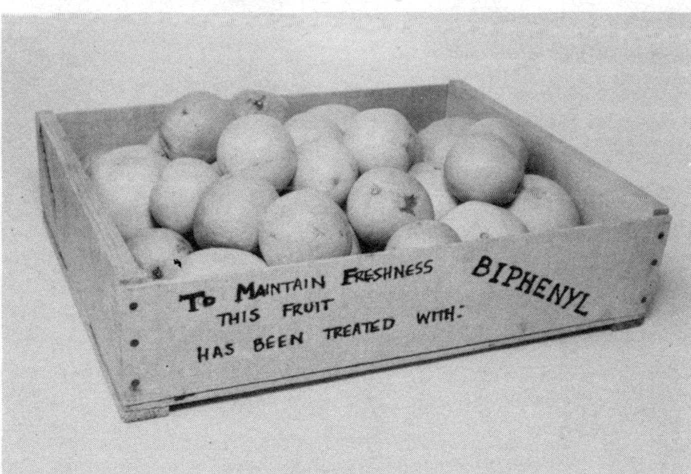

P-2

BIPHENYL ON FRUITS. Biphenyl, a substance used in the embalming process in mortuaries, is also used on fruit as a preservative, to keep it fresh indefinitely. This is only one of thousands of chemicals used in the modern process of preservation of foods.

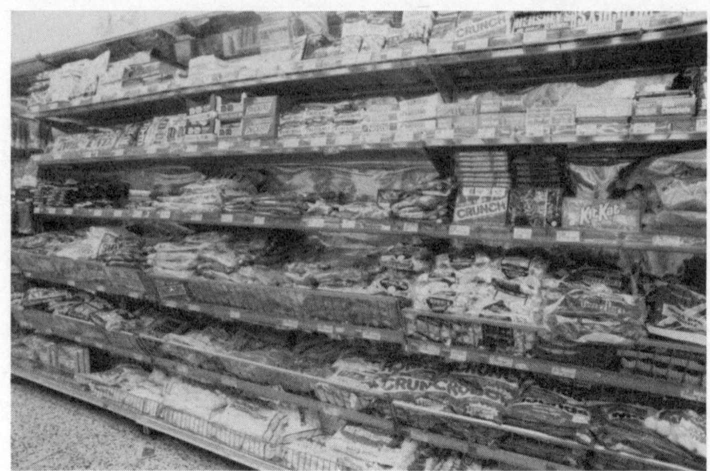

CANDY, CANDY, AS FAR AS THE EYE CAN SEE. Refined sugar causes the teeth to decay, robs one of energy, leaches minerals from the body, causes overweight. Candy has no nutritional value — it is only empty calories.

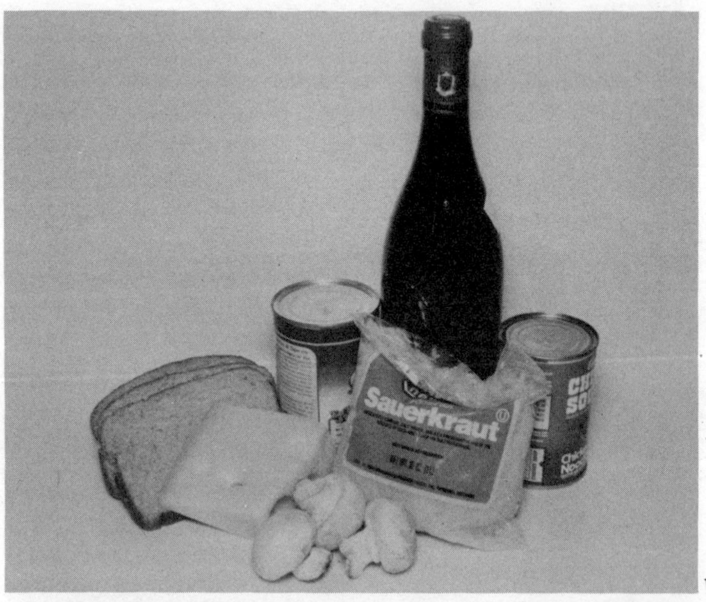

FERMENTED FOODS. Many AIDS patients have Candida Albicans. The main cause of this fungus growth is yeasted foods. A special yeast-free diet and reduced sugar diet is necessary to overcome this condition. Most dry packaged foods and canned foods have yeast in them. Beers and wines, cheeses, breads, sauerkraut, and many canned soups are yeasted or fermented foods and should be avoided. Mushrooms are a fungus; eliminate them from your diet if you have Candida Albicans.

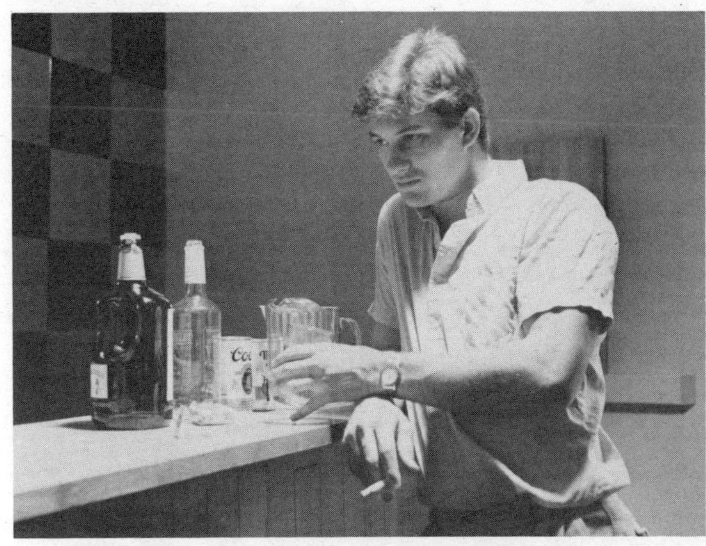

ALCOHOL. Drinking (as well as drug-taking and sexual over-indulgence) has become the "in" thing to do in our time. Alcohol causes psychological and physical addictions and affects the brain cells, the liver, kidneys, and the rest of the body. It becomes an addiction cycle — once one is hooked, it is hard to get off the habit.

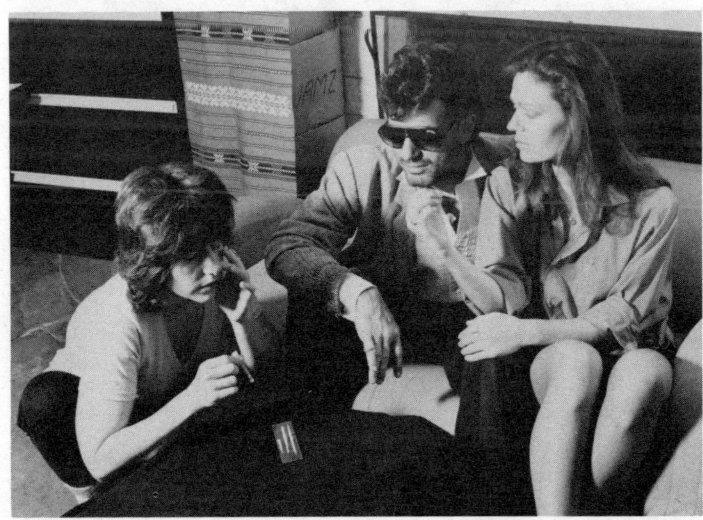

DRUG ABUSE has been closely linked to AIDS in a majority of cases. Cocaine, "recreational" and "designer" drugs, used as sexual stimulants, as well as the inhalation of "poppers" (amyl nitrite and butyl nitrite) are clearly damaging to the immune system.

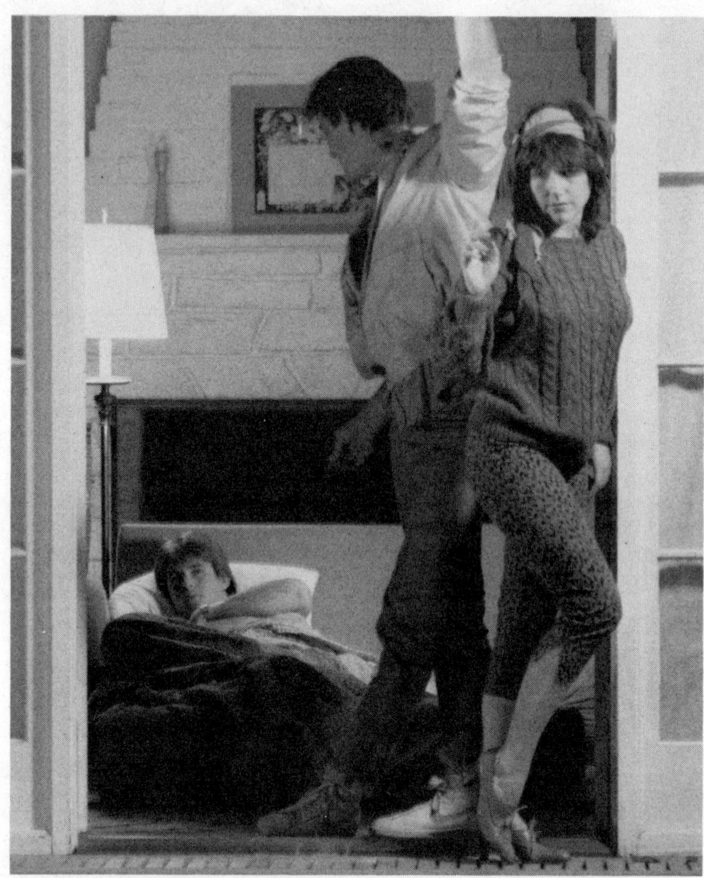

P-7

EXCESSIVE SEXUAL ACTIVITY. There is no question that multiple sex partners, sexual promiscuity and unprotected anal intercourse appear to be the most risky forms of sexual activity in the spread of this disease. A bisexual man with AIDS can pass it on to his female sexual partner.

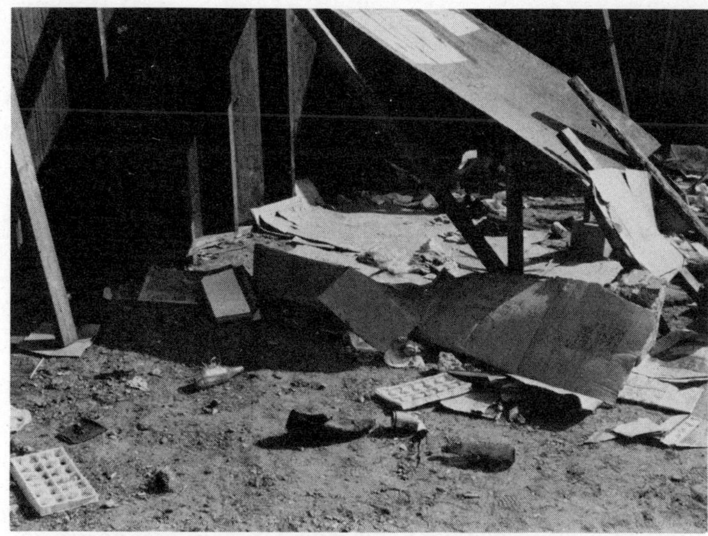

P-8

"HOME." This is the place that someone calls "home." This picture of urban squalor was taken in Los Angeles, but every large city has such places. Belle Glade, Florida, the "AIDS capital of the world," has similar living conditions—poverty, slums, filth—elements that cause disease.

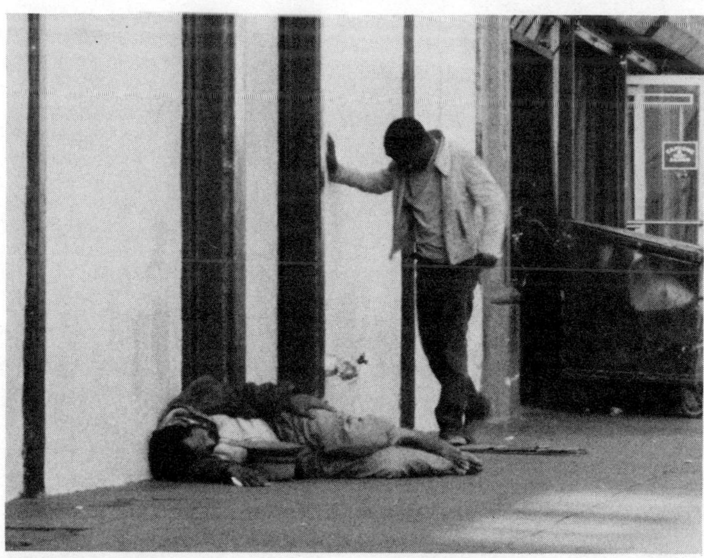

P-9

DRUNKENNESS, IDLENESS, and HOMELESSNESS — by-products of poverty in the city. Such living conditions emanate from many causes: poor early homelife; lack of education, or disinterest in education; alcoholism and other addicting habits; mental illness; society's lack of caring for the homeless.

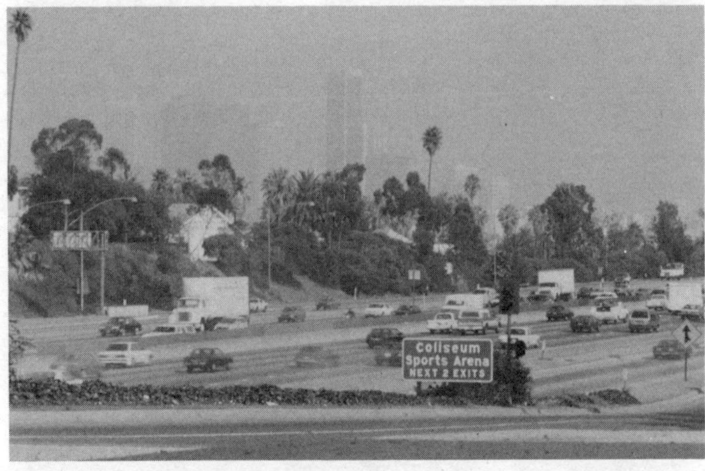

P-10

SMOG. Living in our cities deprives us of the first essential of health—fresh, pure air. Many environmental menaces become endemic (special or particular to one class of persons or district). AIDS thrives in big cities, and environmental pollutants aggravate the threat.

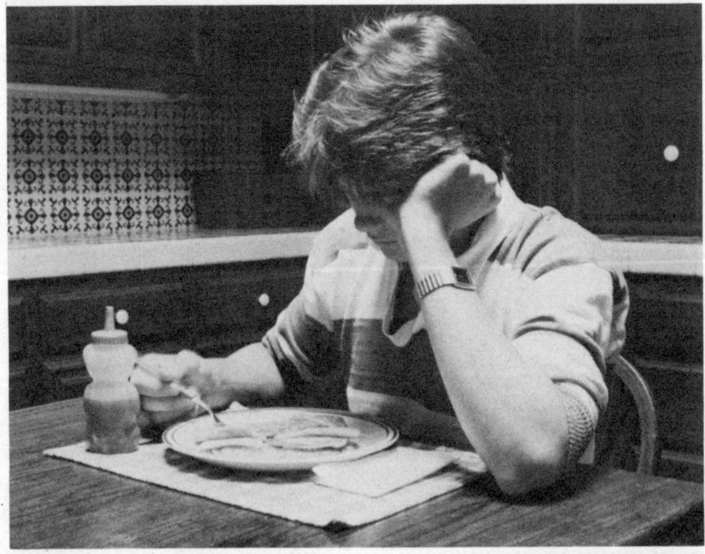

P-11

NO APPETITE. The major beginning symptoms of most diseases are: loss of appetite and sore throat. AIDS is no exception. With AIDS, the symptoms are not the same with all individuals. A person can have one, many, all, or none of the symptoms. In fact, a person can have no symptoms and still be a carrier.

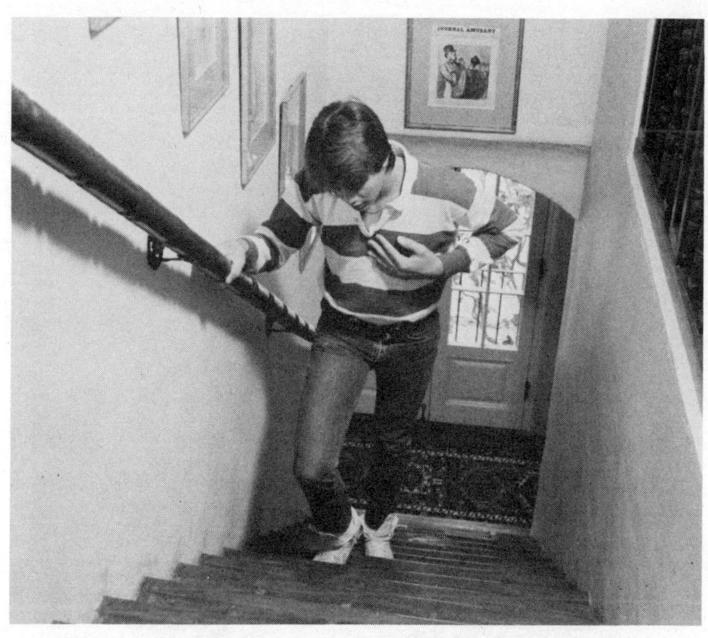

P-12

SHORTNESS OF BREATH. Insufficient respiratory functions can be a symptom of AIDS. Coughing usually accompanies this.

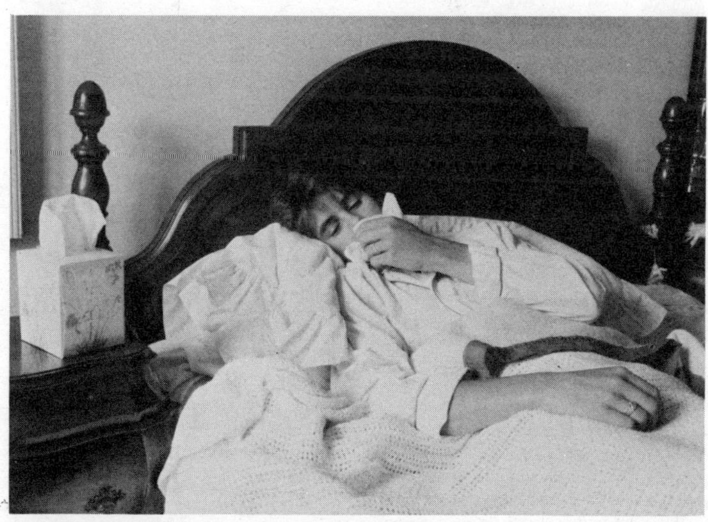

P-13

IN BED WITH FEVER AND COLD. AIDS weakens the immune system, resulting in opportunistic infections, colds, flus, and whatever one comes in contact with.

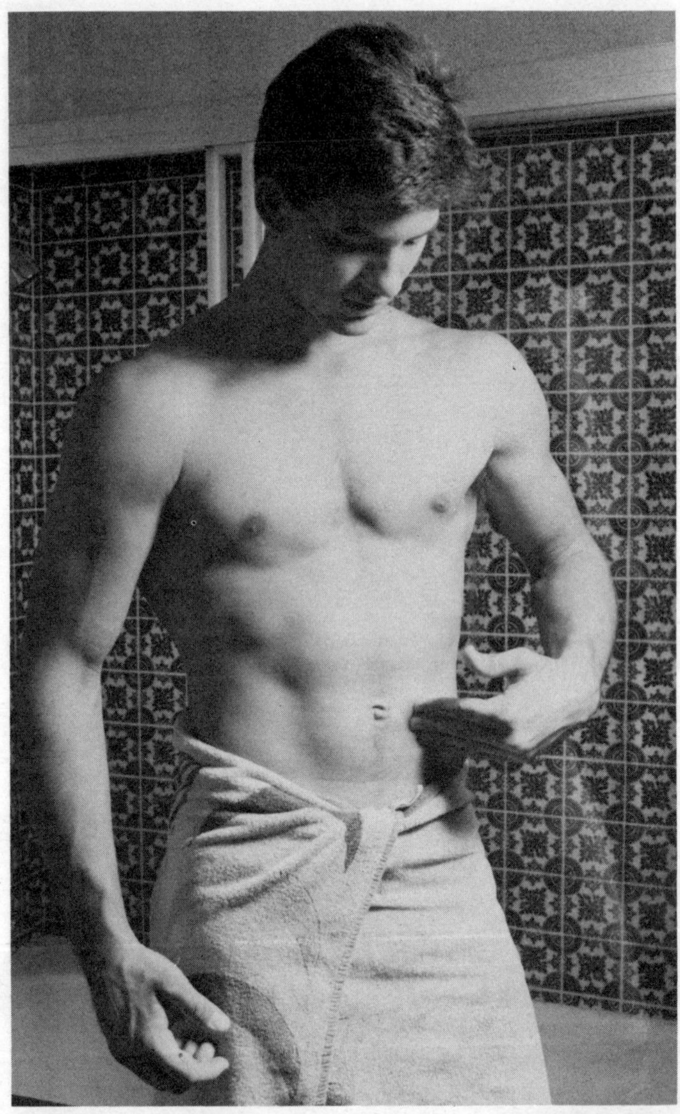

ADRENAL MASSAGE. **This massage, as described in the chapter on Treatment, stimulates the adrenal glands and, if it is done properly, a lowering of the male voice can be heard. The body produces male hormones, which stimulate proper adrenal function; the stimulation gives the male patient strength.**

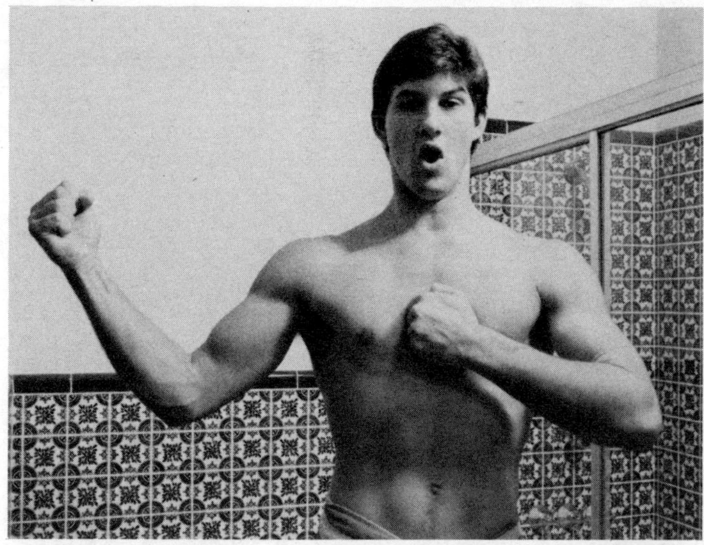

P-15

THUMPING THE THYMUS. Pounding on the sternum of the chest. Gorillas pound on their chests in the same fashion—for it stimulates the thymic function.

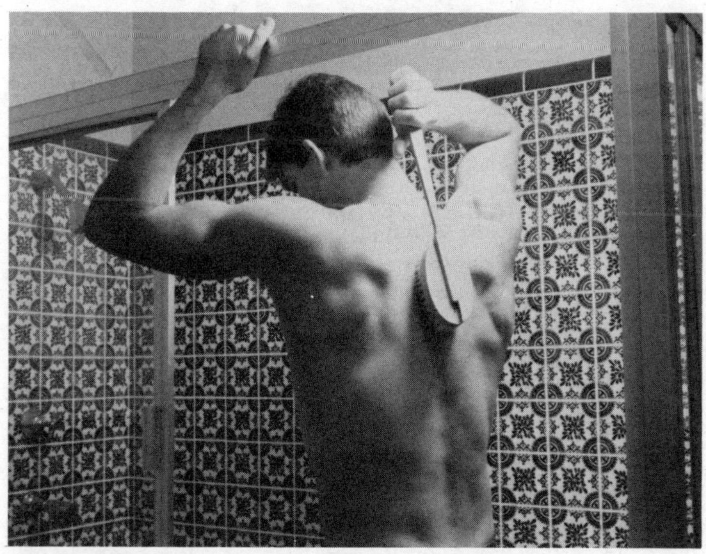

P-16

DRY BRUSH MASSAGE. A self-help mini-acupuncture treatment that stimulates skin response, opens the pores, removes dead skin, and increases circulation, which results in speeded-up metabolism and healing.

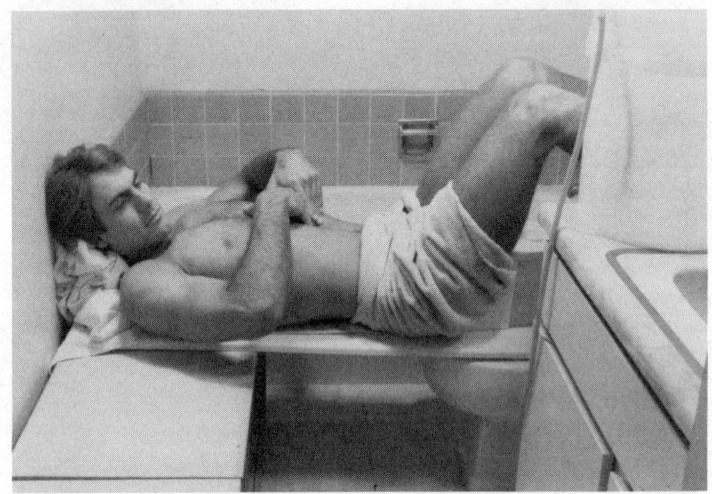

P-17

INTESTINAL CLEANING by non-force gravity flow. First, it cleans the bacteria out of the intestinal system and then it improves the absorption of nutrients. The water goes into the colon by gravity, and washes the toxic residues, poisons, and pathogens out of the system, resulting in the purifying of the blood and, most important, the stimulation of the organs. There are points located in the colon which stimulate the organs. THE SAUNA MUST BE PERFORMED AFTER THIS CLEANING. The reason is that some of the toxins are recirculated back into the system.

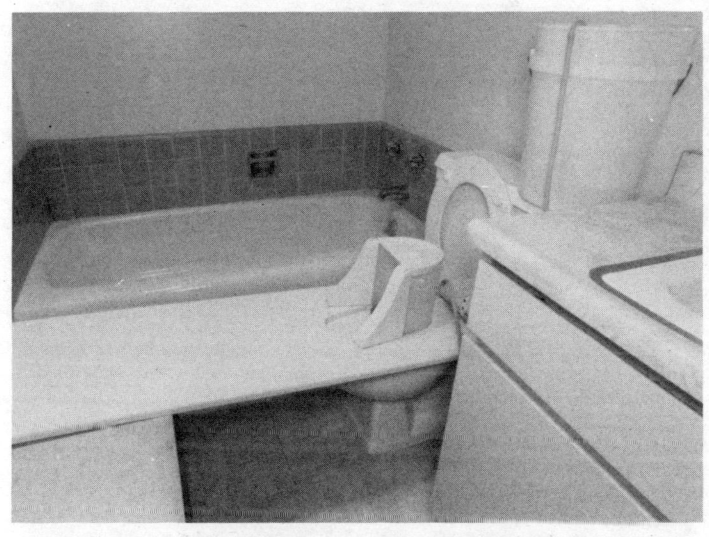

THE COLEMIC BOARD WITH A 5-GALLON BUCKET. This apparatus allows tremendous elimination (up to three pounds at one time) of accumulated, hardened mucus, debris, stool, and toxins. The method is effortless, simple, and inexpensive. Bowel and bladder evacuation and emptying of the bladder can be done at will without removal of the tip of the tube, without turning off the water or getting off the board. It can fit in most bathrooms.

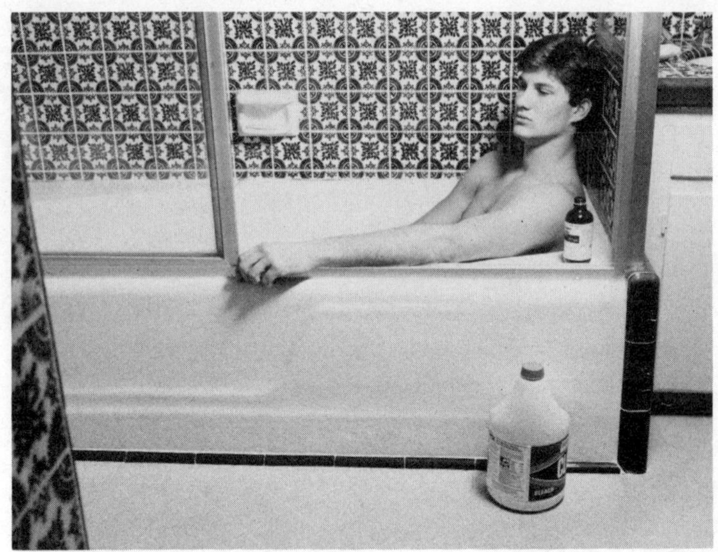

P-19

DETOXIFYING BATHS. Some cancer clinics in Mexico, before cancer treatments, require that their patients detoxify their bodies with superoxide (chlorine bleach) solutions. The patient soaks in this solution in a bathtub.

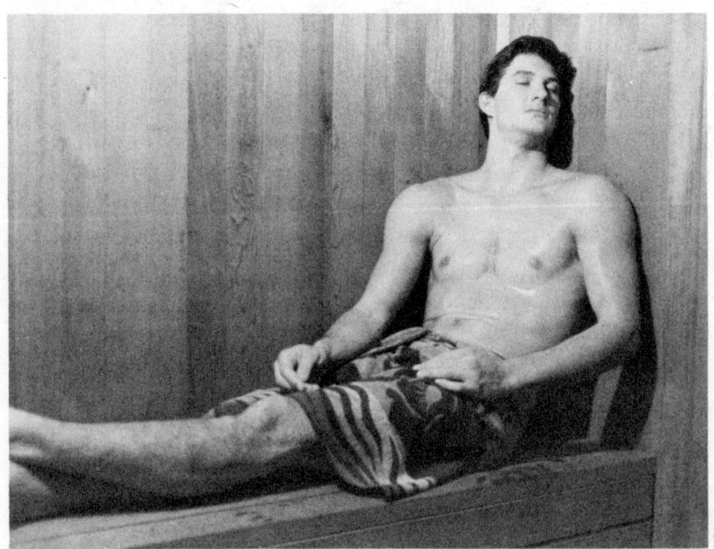

P-20

THE SAUNA increases detoxification by inducing artificial fever. It speeds up circulation and body cell metabolism, thus causing toxic wastes to be expelled through the skin.

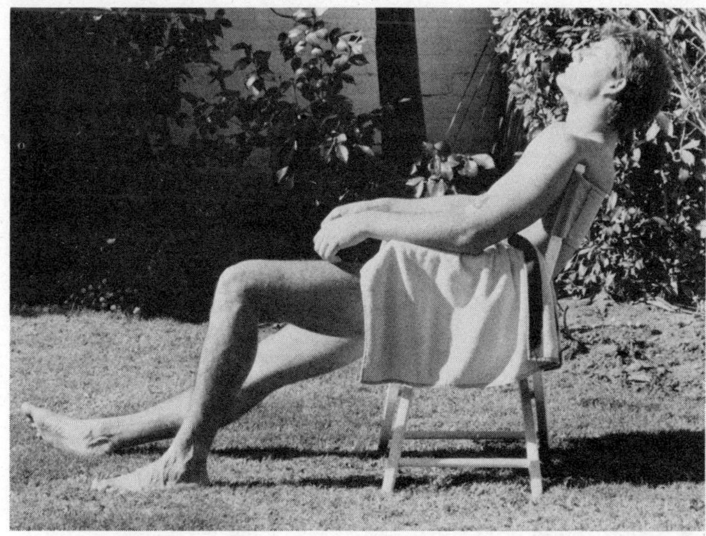

P-21

SUNSHINE ON THE GENITALS. Positioning is very important. The sun's rays should be at a 45° angle (about 4 P.M.). The legs should be bent and spread apart and lifted up toward the abdomen, allowing the sunlight to shine directly on the rectum and genitals.

Before antibiotics were developed, naturopathic doctors were using the sunshine successfully to kill bacteria, germs and pathogens. Sunshine also greatly reduces pain, increases the production of interferon, increases the testosterone level, increases the oxygen to the cells, which strengthens the immune system. This results in lowered blood pressure and helps cancerous conditions and AIDS. The sun's rays may be able to fight against AIDS by increasing the immune response.

There is no evidence, scientifically, that diet alone will eliminate malignant growths. Improving the health of the entire body includes applying sunshine to the skin and using unrefined foods in the diet, which contain plenty of vitamins (C and E), and carotene. When the diet consists of meats, junk foods, etc., especially polysaturated fats, sunshine can be harmful, not helpful, because of free radical formation.

There are two precautions one needs to take with the sun's rays. See the Treatment chapter.

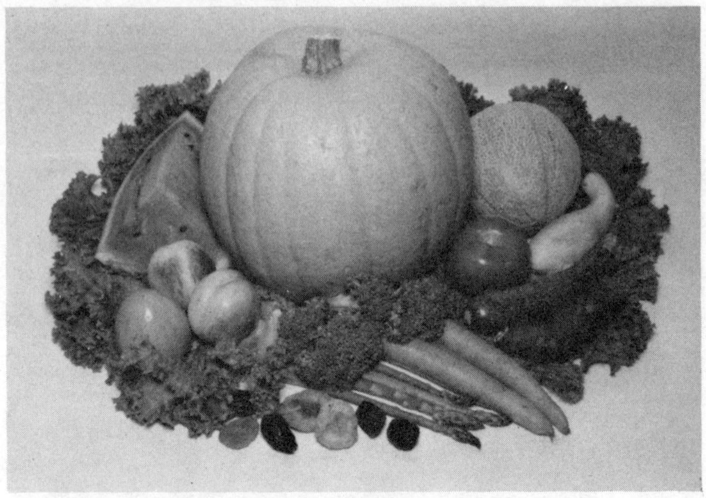

P-22

VITAMIN A. Vegetables and fruits are high sources of Vitamin A—particularly the deeper-colored ones. Use dark green leafy and bright yellow or bright red or orange vegetables especially. Highly recommended: carrots, kale, yams, tomatoes, pumpkin and squash; cantaloupe, persimmons, watermelon. Vitamin A can be as effective as Vitamin C for infections.

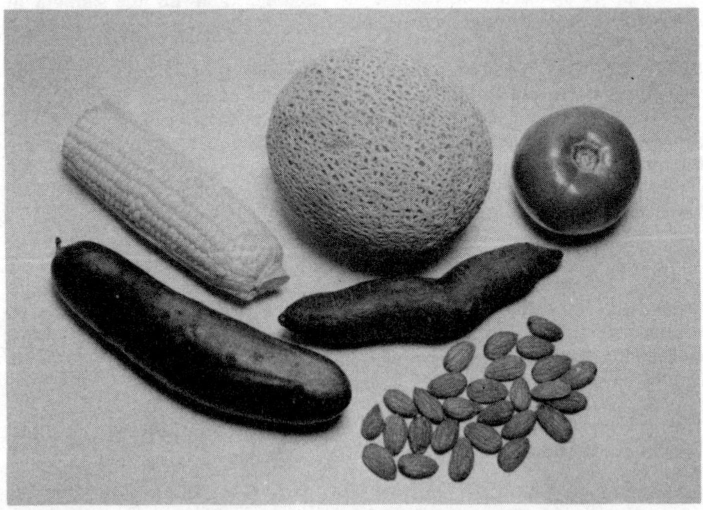

P-23

VITAMIN E. This vitamin is very important for the AIDS patient because it oxygenates the cells. It is found in almonds, seeds (pumpkin and sunflower), cucumbers, corn, sweet potatoes, cantaloupe, tomatoes.

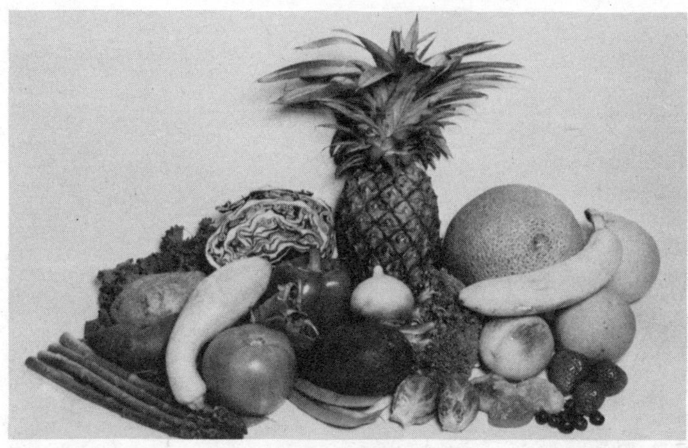

P-24

VITAMIN C. This widely publicized vitamin aids the immune function and is responsible for over 100 bodily processes. The highest sources are citrus fruits (oranges, lemons, grapefruits, limes). In vegetables, look for two colors—red and green. Red has most Vitamin C, so use Mexican red peppers, persimmons and tomatoes. Green is second, so use kale, broccoli, asparagus, parsley, and the green bell pepper (one of the highest sources of Vitamin C).

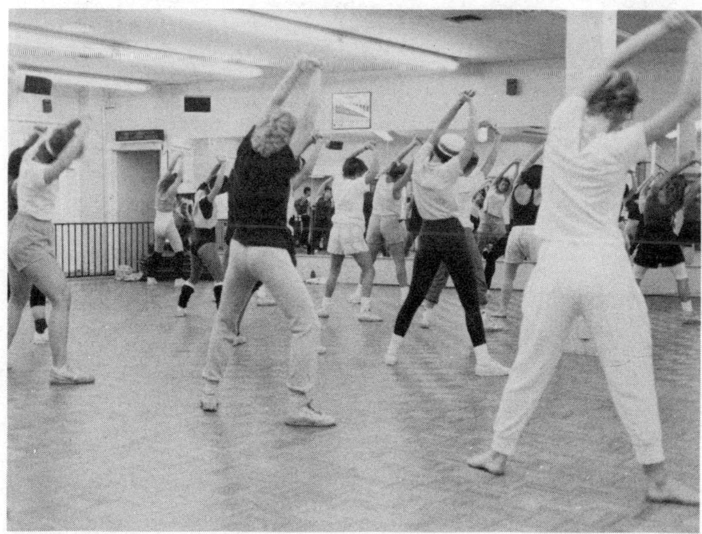

P-25

PHYSICAL EXERCISE. The most important benefits of exercise are to open energy blocks, increase the cardiovascular function, strengthen the heart, improve muscle tone, increase endurance, and produce endorphins, which affect the mental state. Exercise also improves the immune function; it does this by stimulating the organs.

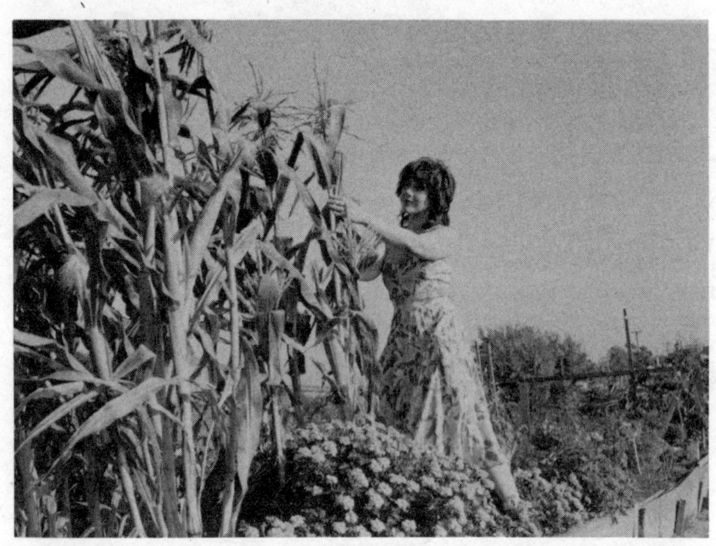

P-26

BACK TO NATURE. Contact with nature is health-inducing. Picking fruits, vegetables and flowers, walking, sunshine, fresh air, swimming in lakes and streams, positive thinking, feeling and speaking, a love of oneself and others, and a moral and civic consciousness—all uplift the person to new heights of health and happiness.

—

EIGHT

—

ACUPUNCTURE AS AN ALTERNATIVE

Acupuncture, an ancient Oriental art of healing, opens up blocked energy fields in the body. The treatment involves a traditional format of looking, hearing, smelling, asking, touching, and listening.

Oriental medicine does not use empirical, scientifically based reasoning; instead, relationships and patterns are studied. Symptoms are clues as to what is going on inside.

Western medicine tends to feel that the structure of an organ determines its function. Simply put, the heart is a muscle which pumps blood. But to the Chinese, the heart governs the entire circulatory system and relates to the mind through the blood's nutrients and circulation.

Modern medicine dissects the whole, and analyzes the parts to the whole. Eastern medicine sees the parts as functioning within the whole.

A story will illustrate this:

A Chinese Master asked a Westerner and an Easterner to tell all about the essence of a goldfish. The Westerner took several pictures, made drawings of every type of goldfish, wrote a thesis on the anatomy, chemistry and physiology of goldfish. He took all this information back to the Chinese Master, saying: "Here is everything you wanted to know about goldfish." The Chinese Master frowned.

The Easterner took the Chinese Master to the edge of the pond, bent down, put his lips to the water. A goldfish swam to the surface's edge, and they kissed.

The Easterner said: "This is the essence of the goldfish."

The Chinese Master approved his answer.

In acupuncture, a *point* means a specific spot on the body surface at which needling is applied. Reactions occur in certain regions or *viscera* (internal organs) so as to produce therapeutic effects. Chinese traditional medicine maintains that all points are capable of both reflecting functional changes of the viscera on the body surface, and passing sensations from the body surface to the viscera. Many diseases are reflected on the interior and exterior of the ear and can be used as diagnostic indicators. Painful spots, pimples or abnormal skin conditions located on acupuncture meridians can also be used as a diagnostic tool.

Meridians are channels or passageways in which energies flow through the body. The Chinese gave a radial, or wrist, pulse to the major energy channels. As each of the channels takes its position in a definite part of the body, and each of the twelve regular channels pertains to and connects with particular organs, the symptoms and signs manifest themselves as disease. Together with the area where they appear, they can serve as a guide to clinical diagnosis.

Take, for example, the liver's function of promoting unrestrained and unobstructed *Chi qi* (or energy), which facilitates the secretion and excretion of bile. Its channel is distributed in the hypochondriac region. Yellow sclera of the eye and hypochrondriac shoulder pain suggest liver disorders. Another example, cough and chest pain, indicates a possible disorder of the lungs; since lungs perform the function of respiration, their channel originates in the chest. Furthermore, tenderness or other abnormal reactions along the area traversed by the channels or at certain points also aids correct diagnosis.

Acupuncture is based on the principle that pathological conditions along channels and collaterals (part of the fourteen total channels) are responsible for the occurrence and transmission of disease. Channels and collaterals are not only the entrances inward for exogenous pathogenic factors; they are also important passages through which disorders impart their influence among organs and tissues of the body.

Of the fourteen meridians in the body, the kidney meridian is extremely important in the treatment of AIDS patients.

In Oriental medicine, the kidneys are responsible for storing a vital essence. This essence is described as our "spark." The kidney energy was so vitally important that two pulse locations were determined and found to exist for the kidneys instead of one.

If this energy (kidney) yang is deficient, we experience extreme fatigue. This yang aspect of the kidneys governs our sexual arousal. An individual can never have too much kidney energy. The yin aspect, *Jing Chi*, governs body development and sexual maturation. Deficiency of kidney essence results in impotence, premature aging and the loss of libido.

The kidney energy is responsible for the production of

marrow that strengthens the bones, enriches the blood and feeds the brain.

Underproduction of marrow leads to arthritis, rickets, dental decay, poor memory, unclear thinking, anxiety, blood anemia, coldness and low-grade fever.

The kidneys control water metabolism. When a deficiency of kidney energy exists, enuresis (frequent urination), night sweats, and edema can result.

The kidneys must hold on to energy that Oriental medicine describes as being ''sent down'' from the lungs. A deficiency of this results in asthma and hyperventilation.

The kidney meridian opens into the ears. A deficiency of kidney energy also results in deafness or tinnitus (ringing in the ears). The kidney energy is also said to govern the anus and urethra, the deficiency resulting in hemorrhoids and arthritis.

BAD HABITS THAT INTERFERE WITH PROPER KIDNEY ENERGY

The consumption of too much salt (overstimulates the kidneys); too much animal protein, especially red meat (has a high salt content, as well as uric acid); alcohol (depletes kidney nutrition); the emotion of fear (damages kidney energy); overwork (drains kidney essence).

In Oriental medicine, a sign of overworked kidneys is swelling and puffiness under the eyes.

It is interesting to note that the aging process is really a description of the loss of kidney energy. When an individual gets old, he develops loss of hearing, brittle bones, poor memory, unclear thinking, loss of libido, coldness, dental decay, and frequent urination.

Acupuncture for the AIDS patient can recirculate and

redistribute energy to deficient organs, resulting in the stimulation of the body's own healing power. Acupuncture can also ease pain, reduce swelling, help to fight infection, and strengthen the whole body. There are never those kinds of side effects that result from the use of powerful drugs.

According to *World Health*, the magazine of the World Health Organization, in 645 cases of acute bacillary dysentery, 90 percent of the patients were cured, using acupuncture, within ten days of examinations. Acupuncture has been used successfully in treating some of the symptoms of heart disease—as well as many other illnesses. It should be tried more with AIDS patients.

NINE

OTHER VIEWPOINTS, OTHER THERAPIES

LAUGHTER AS THERAPY

Norman Cousins wrote a book, *Anatomy of an Illness*, in which he described how he healed himself of a serious collagen disease, largely with this unusual therapy: laughter. He went about it systematically—even rented old films— hilarious comedies from the silent days—to laugh at. It was a concerted effort, and it paid off. This proves how large a part the mental and emotional life of a patient plays in recovery.

Cousins, now on the staff of U.C.L.A., says: "Laughter— along with hope, faith, love, will to live, creativity—can be regarded as an important resource in any strategy of recovery or, indeed, in prompting good health."

In the book, he says that laughter produces chemicals

(hormones called endorphins) that are very beneficial in cases of disease.

Some laughs every day can not only keep the doctor away, but perhaps death itself.

In *Dr. Weisinger's Anger Work-Out Book,* the author, a psychologist, asks the reader if he/she laughs often. If one's daily total of laughs is less than 15, including three bellylaughs—he is "underlaughed."

Laughter is a form of physical and mental fitness that provides lots of accumulated exercise throughout the day.

Mentally, humor is pleasurable and enriching, helps us keep perspective, offers new points of view and unlocks tension.

Physically, research shows that humor aids most—and probably all—major systems of the body, says R. William F. Fry, a psychiatrist at the Stanford University School of Medicine, Stanford, California, and author of three books on humor and health.

A good laugh, Dr. Fry says:

- Gives the heart muscles a good work-out.
- Improves circulation.
- Fills the lungs with oxygen-rich air.
- Clears the respiratory passages.
- Stimulates alertness hormones that stimulate various tissues.
- Alters the brain, diminishing tension in the central nervous system.
- Counteracts fear, anger and depression, all negative emotions linked to physical illness.
- Possibly relieves pain.

Animals do not laugh. Humor is quintessentially human. "It's very important to be thought of as having a good sense of humor," says Clarke McCauley, associate professor of psychology at Bryn Mawr College, Bryn Mawr, PA.

Surprisingly, people in the worst conditions frequently find the most to laugh about. This is a noble aspect of mankind.

Regardless of your situation, if you're not laughing, here's what the experts recommend:

- Know your laughter profile and what makes you laugh.
- Warm up. Start thinking about something funny. If it doesn't seem that funny at first, stay at it.
- Take a humor-meditation break for 5–10 minutes during the tensest part of your day.
- Build a laugh library of favorite humor writers, cartoons, records, tapes, pictures and jokes.
- Be playful with words, images, associations and situations.
- Practice exaggeration for occasional relief.

CANCER IS A LAUGHING MATTER AT THIS CLINIC

At the Wellness Community in Santa Monica, California, cancer patients and their families attend sessions where jokes and laughter are one of the therapies.

Norman Cousins is honorary board chairman. Ken Shapiro is moderator and instigator of the original jokes. Shapiro is playing two roles: that of cancer patient and leader of the group. He is a very funny man who produced and directed the cult favorite "Groove Tube."

It is being discovered that laughter really helps with the recovery process. Harold Benjamin, founder/executive director, states: "The Wellness Community is a place where cancer patients can learn whatever they need to know to fight for their recovery, along with their physicians."

This right idea should be extended to other locations, and to AIDS patients.

PEOPLE WITH AIDS ARE HEALING THEMSELVES WITH LOVE—THE WORK OF LOUISE L. HAY

In Los Angeles, people with AIDS have been attending a weekly workshop facilitated by metaphysical counsellor Louise L. Hay.

The "PWA's" meet in Plummer Park, West Hollywood, to hear Louise Hay advise them how to love themselves, change negative attitudes and thoughts into positive ones, and in that process heal their disease. The sessions offer sharing, loving, and upliftment to all who are receptive.

Because of the widespread fear that permeates the population about this disease, Ms. Hay offers positive direction to a group of people who, up to now, have been without any hope of surviving their illness. Several of her students are now in AIDS remission through using her techniques, in conjunction with healthful nutrition, etc.

Louise Hay said, in an interview: "I began my studies at the Church of Religious Science in New York City, and became a licensed practitioner and minister. I have since studied many other healing modalities. When the doctors said I had cancer, I realized that I was being given the opportunity to practice on myself what I had been teaching to others. A nutritionist and other mental practitioners helped me. Within six months I had no more cancer, and the doctors confirmed it."

This experience helped give Louise Hay the power she has now, and the desire to help persons with AIDS and others. Her message is spreading through workshops and seminars in other cities and even internationally.

She states: "I've created the space where people can come and be honest about themselves."

In her book *You Can Heal Your Life*, she points out that: "Gay men have created a culture that places tremendous emphasis on youth and beauty. While everyone is young to start with, only a few fit the standard of beauty. So much emphasis is placed on the physical appearance of the body that the feelings inside have been totally disregarded. If you are not young and beautiful, it's almost as though you don't count. The person does not count; only the body counts. . . . Because of the ways gay people often treat other gays, for many gay men the experience of getting old is something to dread. It is almost better to die than to get old. And AIDS is a disease that often kills. Too often gay men feel that when they get older, they will be useless and unwanted. It is almost better to destroy themselves first, and many follow a destructive lifestyle."

In his book *Love Your Disease—It's Keeping You Healthy*, John Harrison examines the psychological basis of physical disease. He asks: Why do we decide to be ill? How do we prevent our recovery? How can we heal ourselves? Harrison is a former M.D. who now uses psychology and holistic methods with patients.

Louise Hay's cassette tape *Self-Healing* is calm and reassuring, and has a guided meditation on the reverse side, which can be used daily to advantage.

Louie Nassaney's Story

In August 1986, a conference was held in San Francisco called "Talks on Natural Therapies for Chronic Viral Diseases." Scott J. Gregory was one of the speakers. Many doctors working with natural therapies were among the others, as was Louie Nassaney. He formerly had AIDS and is totally well now. (Doctors like to say "in remission,'' implying that the disease will return, but if a person feels better than he ever felt before—and no longer commits the crimes against his body he once did—why cannot we say he is healed?)

In an interview, Louie Nassaney told us:

''I was diagnosed in May of 1983 as having AIDS. I became an outpatient at U.C.L.A., where the drug interferon was being tested through a government grant. It is a very expensive drug, and I was on it for seven months, in this 'guinea pig' experiment.

''There were many side effects. I had a 100-degree fever for seven months—every day. My injections were on Mondays, Wednesdays, and Fridays, and since the side effects lasted for 24 hours afterwards, I felt a little better only on Sundays. I had to take Tylenol—from 16 to 24 per day—to keep the fever down. My skin became peaked and white; my taste buds were altered; my energy was minimal. I had to sleep from 12 to 15 hours per day.

''At first I was living with roommates, but then I moved back home, to be with my parents, who were very supportive.

''My hearing, sight, touch and coordination were all drastically reduced. The doctors said that since I had only one lesion (Kaposi's sarcoma, on the leg) and it had stabilized, that I should stay on the Interferon.

''But I was not progressing. In the middle of December, 1983, the 18 doctors at U.C.L.A. told me that the Interferon was not working, the lesion was not disappearing. They wanted to use chemotherapy and radiation on me.

''I went to church to pray about it, and after that, I attended church every day to pray. I decided that if I was going to die, it would be naturally, not with a lot of poisons in my body.

''I turned to positive supports of healing. I studied new books. Louise Hay taught me meditation, relaxation, how to love myself, and about spiritual healing energies. I told her I was willing to start changing my thought patterns and lifestyle. Then little miracles started to happen with my body. I went back to the gym for workouts.

"It is a 100% commitment. I see persons with AIDS who hold on to some bad habits, like smoking. You've got to give it all up. I had my share of life in the fast lane, but that is in the past. I have discovered my gift, and I am doing it. I learned that the way to straighten out problems in your life is to start with loving yourself.

"I was fortunate in getting a wonderful support—my family, my church, and Louise Hay and her group.

"I learned to communicate. I am helping people with AIDS now. Although there has been no income from any of this, I now will have a book out. At this point, the title is undecided. It will appeal to the straight community.

"I am on the lecture circuit. I help people whenever I can. On October 7, 1984, the doctors at U.C.L.A. pronounced my disease 'in remission.'

"I used affirmations constantly, such as: 'I am well, I am healed.' I did these out loud; that's more powerful.

"My story was written up in *People* magazine in November 1985, and also in *PM* magazine, the *Los Angeles Times*, the *London Times*, gay publications throughout the U.S., and I was on the *Today* show."

Louie Nassaney has an inspiring story to tell—which shows the power of other therapies—natural and spiritual. A body builder, he is the picture of health, and has a vital message to all Persons With AIDS, other ill persons, to doctors, and the general public. All need to hear this message—that there are other therapies besides drugs —alternative, natural therapies—and THEY WORK.

The quotations from Louise L. Hay in this article are by permission; they are copyrighted by Louise L. Hay.

Also available: "AIDS—A Positive Approach," an audio tape, and "Doors Opening: A Positive Approach to AIDS," a video tape.

CREATIVE VISUALIZATION

(by the Authors)

Exercise in Visualization for Pain Reduction

Sit quietly and breathe deeply. Describe your pain and its intensity—see it as a specific color, shape and dimension. Raise and lift the pain up and out of your body, and physically visualize the pain two inches over your abdomen.

Next, visualize the pain being dissolved by fire, chemicals, a divine power (such as an angel), or any other means that you can imagine. Visualize the pain being dissolved. Say to yourself, "My body is strong and my pain (or my sickness) is weak." Focus your energies on listening to the statements and phrases that you make about yourself. The computer that we call our brain has to be reprogrammed so that what we were taught about ourselves all our lives does not interfere with the healing process.

It has been said that fear is the father of disease and the mother of germs.

Love counteracts fear; it is its antidote.

Exercise in Self-love

Look in the mirror and tell yourself that you love what you see. Do this exercise regularly—daily, or more often.

Exercise in Forgiveness

Make a list of people (past and present) in your life. List the arguments, the hurts and misunderstandings that you remember, where you had negative responses, in thought, feeling, or speech. Acknowledge that you set up the cause and reaped the effects of it.

Tell yourself that you fully forgive yourself and others who sometime in your life hurt you.

Sexual guilt is a strong universal and personal belief. The belief is manifested sometimes in feeling "not good enough."

A positive affirmation is:

"I am a divine, loving expression and victorious over my sexuality and all that I am. I LOVE MYSELF."

This essay on Creative Visualization is, of necessity, only an introduction. If you, the reader, wish to pursue it further, books, tapes, and seminars are available for you to explore it more deeply. But this outline does give you a start, and the most important part is to DO IT. Our love goes out to you in your successful manifestation of health and happiness, through Creative Visualization, and all our other natural therapies, outlined in this book.

Recommended: *Creative Visualization* **by Shakti Gawain is an inspirational bestseller that has led thousands of persons to the fulfillment of their desires through the Art of Mental Energy and Affirmation. (Bantam New Age Books.)**

THE TREE OF TOXEMIA
A Graphic Depiction of Diseases and their Causes

Dr. John H. Tilden's book *Toxemia Explained* was published in 1926. For the first time, a formal theory of diseases and their universal cause had been advanced. At the time, Dr. Tilden was 75 and had been in the health movement for more than 50 years. Those who call themselves Natural Hygienists had been attributing diseases to self-poisoning

THE TREE OF TOXEMIA

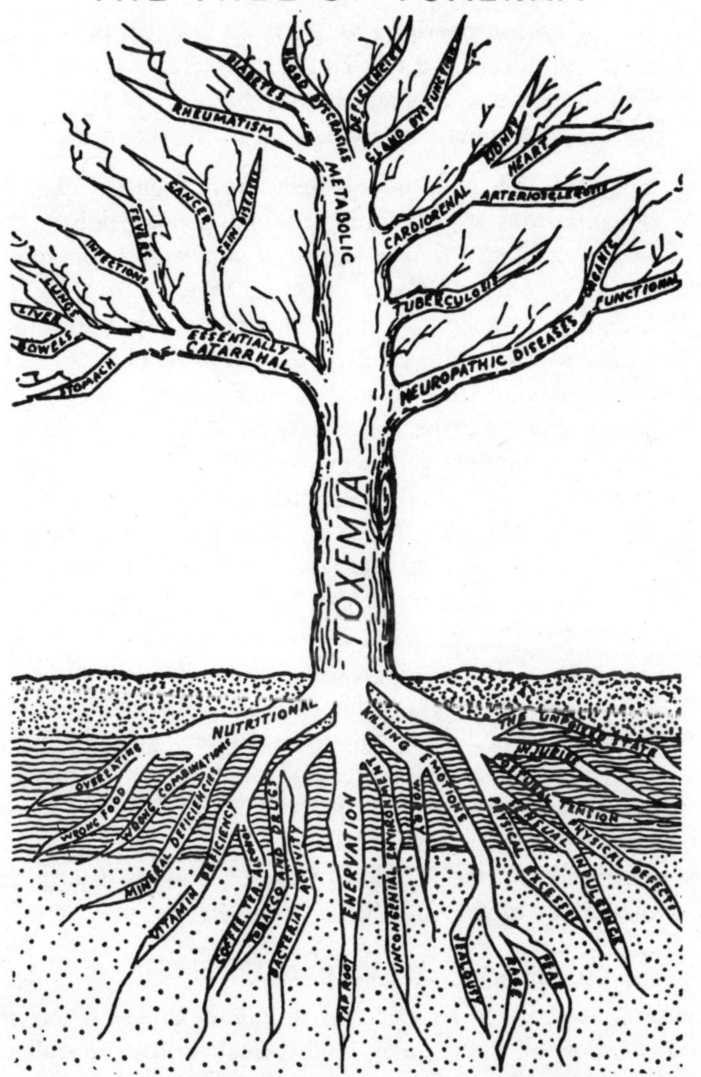

A GRAPHIC ILLUSTRATION OF THE THEORY OF TOXEMIA AS FORMULATED BY J. H. TILDEN, M.D., WHICH SHOWS HOW DISEASE IS BUILT BY UNNATURAL LIVING HABITS.

of the body for nearly 100 years before he published *Toxemia Explained*, but Dr. Tilden (an M.D.) was the first to give the statements a substantive basis.

Basically, toxemia causes disease in this manner:

1. The body becomes intoxicated* from ingested exogenous poisons or uneliminated endogenous poisonous wastes or both. *(*The meaning of intoxicate in pathology is "to poison.")*
2. Intoxication occurs because the body has a lowered ability to eliminate, due to enervating influences, i.e., stress, devitalizing poisons, insufficient sleep, etc. It cannot generate the necessary nerve energy to cope with the eliminative needs—or the ingestion of poisons exceeds the body's eliminative capacities.
3. The exhaustion of life's vital fund of nerve energy due to overwork, physical excesses, overeating, deficiencies of nutrients, draining emotions, etc., per the roots as labelled in the chart.
4. Because of the saturation of blood and tissues with toxic materials, severe interference with bodily functions occur and body integrity is threatened. To cope with the dire situation, the body initiates an extraordinary emergency cleansing/detoxification crisis. The manner in which the body conducts the expulsion of toxic materials and the location of the exit points determine the names of the so-called afflictions.

Thus it can be seen that diseases are massive bodily efforts to redirect its energies to an emergency act of purification of tissues and fluids. Such crises are called acute diseases.

If toxic practices are chronic, the toxic condition of the body becomes chronic and organic damage is bound to result. When organic damage occurs, degeneration has occurred and the resulting ailments are said to be degenerative. Acute diseases are constructive in that they cleanse and repair the body, but degenerative diseases are destructive, for they involve the derangement of faculties. Fevers, colds, acne, boils, asthma and canker sores are constructive in that they endeavor to free the body of encumbering toxins and repair damages. Cancer, arthritis, diabetes, arteriosclerosis and multiple sclerosis may be termed degenerative diseases, for they represent the actual destruction of faculties.

The answer to toxemia is to detoxify the body by fasting and to keep it pure by adopting non-toxic eating and living practices.

T. C. FRY

PRESIDENT, *College of Life Science*, AUSTIN, TEXAS

(Note: Harvey and Marilyn Diamond, authors of the bestselling book *Fit for Life*, took this course in health before writing their remarkable book that is helping to change the nation's concepts about health and disease, diet and weight loss.)

NEURO-LINGUISTIC PROGRAMMING, "REFRAMING," and ANTHONY ROBBINS

"N-L-P," a new psychological tool, especially its technique of "reframing," is having a great impact on health.

This means taking negative emotions and destructive thought patterns and changing the way we perceive people and situations. It involves discarding the negative viewpoint, finding something positive about the situation, and building it up.

Anthony Robbins, leader of seminars on Neuro-Linguistic

Programming, teaches this. He is the author of the best-selling book *Unlimited Power* (Simon & Schuster), on this dynamic new technique. In the book, he gives this example:

"A boy named Stanley was born blind. When he asked his mother why he was blind, she did not give him a reply that would create a self-image of himself as 'victim.' Instead, she replied: 'I don't know, but I do know that you can do anything anyone else can do, and you are as good as anybody else. What others can see with their eyes, you can see with your hands.' He became a great and famous adult. Throughout his life, he continued to use this 'reframing' tool."

Whatever the circumstance, handicap, negative emotion or situation, it can be turned into an *advantage*.

Disease works this way also, because it shows us that we have done something or allowed something to be done to our bodies, resulting in an unhealthy state. This can be reframed because: firstly, it is a re-learning process, and, secondly, if we learn what we need to do to get well, and do so, then we can help others to do the same.

SOME NEW ASPECTS ON AIDS

"There is no historical precedent for believing that a single infectious agent is capable of abolishing a normal immune system."

—ARTHUR J. AMMANN, M.D.,
UNIVERSITY OF CALIFORNIA SCHOOL OF MEDICINE,
SAN FRANCISCO, CA, 1984.

''The AIDS epidemic will produce an enormous and frightening effect on world health that public health officials may be relatively powerless to contain.''

—DR. WILLIAM A. HASELTINE,
AIDS RESEARCH, HARVARD MEDICAL SCHOOL

''In many areas, the number of persons infected with the AIDS virus is at least one hundred times greater than the reported cases of AIDS.''

DR. JAMES CURRAN,
CENTERS FOR DISEASE CONTROL

''The AIDS virus shows every sign of being just as deadly as the plague during the Middle Ages. We are on a crash course with reality. . . . The alarm must be sounded, loudly and persuasively. If it is not, the conclusion is inescapable: millions may die.''

''There is a growing reservoir of infection among urban prostitutes, and men who utilize their services run the risk of infection.''

''The rapidly growing number of pediatric AIDS cases is one of the most tragic aspects of the AIDS crisis. For infected parents to consider a pregnancy is to put the mother and unborn infant in a life-threatening situation.''

''. . . The day when there are millions of young, single infected people in America may soon be upon us. . . . Will the next decade or two witness a serious rollback of the era of permissiveness which we have been experiencing since the middle of the 1960s?''

DR. J. A. SLAFF,
THE AIDS EPIDEMIC (Warner Books)

An article in *The Saturday Evening Post* (October, 1986) is entitled "Did 'Dr. X' Cure His Own AIDS?" It is written by Editor and M.D. Cory SerVaas. Two of the substances the doctor used were lysine and zinc—and we have been recommending them in this book. He does not reveal his name, but interested persons can contact the magazine.

"Clinicians from Boston to San Francisco now realize that AIDS is a hydra-headed complex of diseases, embracing not only the narrow syndrome first described, but many more infections and cancers."

—Wall Street Journal, May 30, 1986.

This, too, has been our opinion since 1985.

It is being realized that AIDS is a multi-faceted disease; therefore, it causes a multi-faceted controversy.

Since the beginning of the AIDS epidemic, a connection between drugs and the syndrome was apparent. Other factors must be questioned, such as: Iatrogenic causes (medically-induced); anal hydrogenated fat lubricants* (see below); poor nutrition and sanitation; parasites from "opportunistic" infections, bacteria and fungi; multi-viral infections; and fluoridated drinking water.

*Lawrence Burton, Ph.D., asked: "Could it be that these lubricants, commonly used by homosexuals in anal intercourse, are being absorbed into their systems, and causing immune depression?" Dr. Burton experimented by using these fats with mice (given to them to eat, and also applied anally). He produced AIDS-like symptoms, and ten out of twelve of the mice died.

Studies have also been done of polysaturated fats, taken orally as foods. The result was cancers, immune functions destroyed, and the inhibition of the production of prostaglandins in the body, which help in the manufacture of T-cells.

NEW LIGHT ON AIDS—
THE HOMEOPATHIC PERSPECTIVE

Dana Ullman is an author, publisher, and educator whose specialty is homeopathic medicine. He is president of the Foundation for Homeopathic Research in Berkeley, California. He presents some provocative ideas on AIDS, on disease and on health. His statements are within quotation marks.

"One of the major myths about AIDS is that *healthy* people get it. That's a destructive myth; it's not true. Healthy people do not 'get' AIDS. It's difficult to get the disease. People who develop AIDS are individuals who usually have had significant and repeated stress to their immune systems."

(He goes on to say that the HIV virus is actually a weak virus, and a healthy body is or should be strong enough to deal with it, as well as other viruses or bacteria.)

"Researchers have noted that poor nutrition, repeated bacterial infections, certain viral infections, unsafe sex practices, exposure to toxic substances, and use of certain recreational drugs can weaken immune response.

"I find it ironic that authorities have singled out these drugs while completely ignoring various commonly used therapeutic drugs which have suppressive effects on the immune system, as well as on other parts of a person's defense system.

"There is now some evidence that strongly suggests that penicillin, and possibly other antibiotics, may be a co-factor to the development of AIDS. [Mentions the *Journal of The American Medical Association*.] It is widely recognized that penicillin *does* decrease white blood cells. . . . It may inhibit the body's own defenses in other ways as well. More specifically, we find that, in toxic doses, ANTIBIOTICS, INCLUDING PENICILLIN, REDUCE OUR BODY'S ABILITY TO DEFEND ITSELF AGAINST SPECIFIC INFECTION.

"They also, in overdose, reduce the bacteria in our intestines that are important for assimilating food. The body, then, doesn't assimilate food as well, resulting in insufficient nourishment, which also weakens the defenses.

"It is startling to learn that many of the major symptoms of AIDS are very similar to the symptoms that penicillin is known to cause, in overdose, or simply to those people who are allergic to the drug. Besides poor absorption of food and gradual loss of weight, penicillin is known to lead to decreases in white blood cells, increased susceptibility to infection, skin rash, fever and chills, neurological problems, and other similar symptoms of AIDS.

"I must be clear in saying that antibiotics such as penicillin do not *cause* AIDS, but it is my assumption that if a person is infected with the HTLV-III virus [subsequently renamed HIV] at the same time that the defense system has been stressed by the taking of significant doses of penicillin, the chances of getting the disease may be increased.

"It's important that a person, especially a person in the so-called high-risk group, who has an infection—for instance, strep throat, or an ear infection, or pneumonia—should know he does *not* have to run to the doctor to take antibiotics. . . . The problem that we have created is that we've used penicillin like candy, weakening our defense systems."

Ullman goes on to point out that many medicines "have been abandoned because they were found to cause more harm than good. . . . For many decades people assumed they were basically harmless . . . now we're finding that they are *not* harmless. They can create various strains of bacteria which are resistant to the particular antibiotic, and they can create various other side effects which can be detrimental to general health."

Dana Ullman quotes the AIDS campaign slogan—and

(Quotations reprinted, with permission, from *The Sentinel,* San Francisco, California, December 5, 1985. Interview by Ken Coupland.)

we heartily agree—and this is what our book is all about—''THE BEST PREVENTION IS EDUCATION.'' There is a greater disease than AIDS, and that is ignorance. EDUCATE—AND CONQUER AIDS NOW!

A LETTER FROM DR. NORMAN W. WALKER TO BIANCA LEONARDO

Dear Dr. Leonardo:

Thank you for the copy of your book, *Cancer and Other Diseases Caused by Meat Consumption—Here's the Evidence*. I hope you will sell a million of these.

As you no doubt know, I am not in favor of meat, even at its best, as a source of protein. In addition, there is the esthetic angle, or rather, the lack thereof.

People fail to realize that the body needs only an average of three or four ounces of protein replenishment a day. Nitrogen is its important ingredient. Where do we get it?

Almighty God KNEW how much we need and its best regular source, namely, the AIR WE BREATHE! It contains 75% nitrogen and we get a mouthful, or nose-full, every breath! Raw vegetables, fruits and sprouted seeds supply the balance.

I again thank you for your book and for the message you expound.

With my kindest regards and best wishes,

Sincerely yours,

N. W. Walker, M.D., D.O., D.C., N.D., D.Sc., Ph.D.

Note by Bianca Leonardo: This precious man—brilliant, good, kind, humane, selfless, wise—left this plane on June 6, 1985, at age 109. He was one of a kind. We honor him by trying to live as he did.

DR. NORMAN WALKER'S VIEWPOINT ON COLON HEALTH RELATED TO GENERAL HEALTH

Pioneer Dr. Walker has left us a heritage of many books which explain his discoveries. One of them is: *Colon Health: The Key to a Vibrant Life*. We strongly recommend discovering this book and practicing his precepts to better health through natural methods. He discusses many organs and parts of the body. Quoting briefly:

"(Seeing) the proximity of the prostate gland to the rectum, you will appreciate the need for colon irrigations to prevent the excessive accumulation of feces and other waste matter in the region of the anus and the rectum. Once this area becomes clogged and its contents magnified, the pressure against the prostate can, and usually does, cause either prostate or testicle trouble.

"There comes to mind a case of an Italian laborer whose testicles were enlarged very nearly to the size of a rugby football and his prostate also inflamed. . . . He was afraid to go to a medical doctor. I was able to induce him to take a dozen colon irrigations. In the course of two or three months he appeared on his own volition for another dozen irrigations. In about 18 months his testicles were almost normal and his prostate trouble had vanished."

In another case from his files, a woman with lumps over most of her body was scheduled for cancer surgery the next morning. When she discovered this, she dressed and fled the hospital. She asked Dr. Walker for advice, which was: colonics and consuming much fresh vegetable juice, and raw fresh fruits and vegetables, instead of the orthodox meals.

The result was: every single lump disappeared from her body, and that without any surgery—totally naturally.

THE PLANETARY PROBLEM AND NEW HOPE

It has been said that AIDS has the potential of ending America as we know it by the next century. This makes AIDS one of the most important diseases of our age. Here is the vital question: Is AIDS polluting humanity's bloodstream?

It is a crucial time—time for a new breakthrough! And alternative, natural therapies ARE that breakthrough.

Our aim in this book was and is to help persons in a sickened state do something for themselves in healing —to take responsibility for their disease. Simply, AIDS is caused by what certain individuals do to themselves, and also what they allow others to do to them. (Children with AIDS are helpless, innocent victims of others' mistakes.)

In this book and in "C.A.N.! UPDATE," our new newsletter, our aim is to inspire the reader to learn more natural, healthful ways of living and encourage him to change any destructive lifestyle he might be following. People must learn what proper nutrition is, practice it, and follow the other natural laws of living—resulting in a harmonious, happy, healthy life—a rarity these days!

We hope to help the person with AIDS cope with and overcome the fear this disease generates—rather than leaving him helpless and hopeless. We wish to influence the person with AIDS to improve the quality of his life. Prevention must be practiced and alternative, natural therapies must be tried.

Drugs do not heal the body; it heals itself. Sometimes it needs outside help, but drugs are not that help.

Most persons are skeptical about natural treatments because they get little publicity, while new drugs and other allopathic measures get the full cooperation of the government, the universities, business, and the media. There are no huge profits to be made in alternate therapies. For them to be accepted as effective and legitimate, there is much work to be done. They must be given a real opportunity to prove themselves in a controlled environment. But they suffer from a news "blackout" by the media. Material medicine has a virtual monopoly on news exposure, at present.

Tax monies are used on every level of government for AIDS research. But AIDS is not just one disease, but a combination. Therefore, there will never be merely one cure, like the "miracle" drug or vaccine the drug companies are searching for.

AIDS HAS BROUGHT A CRISIS TO HUMANITY, BUT ALSO AN OPPORTUNITY. Now we can look in another direction for health and healing, besides drugs.

This book, the first of its kind (natural therapies applied to AIDS), is a pioneer, and points the way for mankind. Please spread the news in whatever way you can—tell another about the book, buy copies for gifts, and subscribe to the newsletter, "C.A.N.! UPDATE." We thank you very much for being on our team that is striving to help humanity.

There is still time. Instead of our heading into a long night of a new "dark ages," we can walk toward the light of a new "Golden Age." It is up to all of us to choose which way we, and mankind, shall go.

TEN

A HISTORY OF AIDS

The examination of the history of AIDS shows that one or more diseases commonly occur in AIDS and the signs and symptoms produced by these different diseases can vary tremendously in AIDS patients. For instance, some people with AIDS may have one or more "opportunistic infections," each produced by a different microbe. Some AIDS victims have cancer tumors, particularly a rare form of cancer known as Kaposi's sarcoma. Some people with AIDS have both infections and cancer.

It is interesting to note that cancer patients receiving chemotherapy, and patients with hepatitis, infectious mononucleosis and other diseases, show immunosuppression similar to that in AIDS patients.

AIDS is the only infectious disease in medical history in which age limits for diagnosis have been established.

According to the Centers for Disease Control (CDC) criteria, all persons older than 65 with cancer are excluded from the diagnosis of AIDS. Patients taking immunosuppressive drugs and cancer chemotherapy are also excluded. It would seem that these would be high-risk groups for AIDS; nevertheless, these two groups are excluded from the diagnosis.

Is it possible that medical scientists may unwittingly be producing a monster by the widespread use of chemotherapy, antibiotics, and radiation? Is it possible that the cancer microbe is made more aggressive, not only by other invading microbes, but also by chemotherapeutic drugs, prescribed for their eradication? Have the modern treatment methods changed the nature of the cancer microbe, and allowed it to produce a different kind of disease such as AIDS? **Although doctors realize a healthy immune system is the body's best defense against AIDS, it is ironic to realize that treatment, such as chemotherapy, often injures the immune system.**

The AIDS epidemic has already encouraged many people to improve the quality of their lives and improve their personal relations. For some people who have lovers and friends with AIDS, the epidemic has taught them the meaning of life—to live and love, and care more deeply.

In 1872, a Hungarian doctor named Moriz Kohn (who changed his name to Moriz Kaposi) reported on the study of five patients with tumors; all these men were between the ages of 40 and 60, and all had come to his dermatology clinic in Vienna, Austria.

He described the skin disease as being rapidly lethal, with death occurring within two or three years. Today, most physicians consider "classic" Kaposi's sarcoma the least life-threatening form of cancer.

Kaposi was also aware that Kaposi's sarcoma tumors could also be found inside the body. More than a century after the discovery of the disease, the cause of Kaposi's sarcoma remains a mystery. There is one thing that is new and certain about this disease. Kaposi's sarcoma is occurring with tremendous frequency among homosexual men in New York City, Los Angeles, San Francisco, and other American cities.

For the first time in medical history, a sexually transmitted microbe is thought to be a possible cause of this type of cancer. Kaposi would have been surprised by the current idea that Kaposi's sarcoma might be infectious or even contagious. At the time he discovered the disease (1872), microbes were not considered to be a cause of any infectious disease. At this point, the reader should be asking: Is a cancer contagious? Kaposi's sarcoma has always been a peculiar form of cancer. Some tumors of Kaposi's sarcoma may be persistent for decades and miraculously vanish as fast as they appear.

It is interesting to note that Andrew Harwood, *et al.* (1979), in Toronto, Canada, concluded that ''the increased incidence of Kaposi's sarcoma in renal transplant recipients suggests that immunosuppression may be an important factor in the development of the disease.'' When immunosuppressive drugs were discontinued, the tumors of Kaposi's sarcoma often diminished in size or disappeared.

There has always been controversy as to whether Kaposi's sarcoma is a malignant or benign form of cancer. It has been suggested by some scientific investigators that Kaposi's is not cancer, but rather an infection, perhaps due to a microbe.

Some pathologists even question whether Kaposi's sarcoma is a ''true'' virus. One of the most distressing features of Kaposi's sarcoma is that more than one-third of the people who contract this form of cancer will develop some other form of cancer. One-third of all patients diagnosed as having AIDS either have, or will develop, a malignant cancer such as Kaposi's. For this reason, AIDS must be considered a ''pre-cancerous'' disease as well as a symptomatic illness.

In central Africa, where the AIDS virus is endemic, a similar form of the virus is found in the green monkey. One theory is that the virus is spread to man by contact with these green monkeys, by bites or scratches, by eating them or through bestiality. (See *The AIDS Cover-up?* by Gene Antonio, Ignatins Press, p. 1.) Another possible factor in the spread of AIDS is by contaminated needles used in the rituals of scarification (putting decorative scars on the body). In the African epidemic, men and women are victims in equal numbers. Promiscuous sex and poor sanitation are other factors.

Belle Glade, Florida, only 49 miles from posh Palm Beach, has been called a world-class ghetto. It is a squalid, mosquito-infested shanty town, where most of the dilapidated houses lack cooking facilities and running water, and where children run barefoot through broken bottles and rat droppings in the streets.

The population is only 20,000, but Belle Glade is gaining notoriety as the unofficial AIDS capital of the world. Between 1982 and 1985, forty-six cases have been reported, a per capita incidence about three times that of New York and San Francisco. Twenty-three of the victims were known to have belonged to one of several high-risk groups, and one woman contracted the disease from her husband, an intravenous drug user. The other 22 cases did not seem to fall into any high-risk category, although 13 were immigrants from Haiti (where the disease is well established).

The pattern of the infections in Belle Glade is unlike that anywhere else in the U.S.—and that could have a grave implication for non-drug-using heterosexuals. At least, that is the controversial view of Mark Whiteside of the Institute of Tropical Medicine in North Miami. He believes the high incidence of AIDS in Belle Glade—or in central Africa for that matter—cannot be explained unless environmental factors, especially mosquito infection, are considered. "I don't buy the arguments that AIDS is caused by one virus that travels slowly through the blood, or by sexual contact," says Whiteside. "Every major epidemic in history has been linked to environmental factors." But few AIDS researchers accept his theory.

The AIDS epidemic officially began in America in June, 1981. Many cases reported in medical literature suggest that some people in other parts of the world acquired AIDS-like illnesses before that time.

Early in 1985, most Americans had become aware of AIDS, conscious of a trickle of news about a new disease that was threatening homosexuals and drug addicts. AIDS, the experts said, was spreading rapidly. The number of cases was increasing geometrically, doubling every ten months.

It was the shocking news of actor Rock Hudson's illness that finally catapulted AIDS out of the closet, transforming it overnight from someone else's problem, a "gay plague," to a cause of international alarm.

"NO ONE IS SAFE FROM AIDS," on the cover of *Life* magazine in July, 1985, resulted in a series of factual omissions and hazy conclusions, leading to much misinformation spreading to other media. The most common problem found in early reporting was the lack of coordinated, specifically correct data. There were many contradictions and often theories were reported as facts.

The disease was often said to be transmitted by "intimate sexual contact or an exchange of bodily fluids.'' In another statement, ''much remains unknown about how the AIDS virus spreads.'' And finally, ''no description of AIDS is really complete without reference to the breakage of the rectal lining from anal intercourse . . . this is probably how the majority of the cases have been transmitted so far. . . .''—a fact that underlines the remoteness of the AIDS risk from the experience of most people. Now ''NO ONE IS SAFE''???

Similarly, reporters rarely point out the correlation between AIDS risks and people who are extremely promiscuous (hundreds of sex partners).

In May, 1983, syndicated columnist Patrick Buchanan (former Director of Communications at the White House) wrote that ''homosexuals have declared war upon nature, and now nature is exacting an awful retribution.''

Suddenly AIDS was front-page news on the TV talk shows. There seemed to be no end to the reports.

Item: ''Rock Hudson was flown home today from Paris, France, and was transferred on a stretcher to a waiting helicopter, which took him from Los Angeles International Airport to UCLA's Medical Center in Westwood for further medical treatment. . . .''

Item: ''Lester Maddox, former Governor of Georgia, started undergoing tests out of fear that he might have received the microbe that causes AIDS from contaminated blood serum prescribed by a controversial cancer clinic in the Bahamas. . . .''

Item: ''In Kokomo, Indiana, today, a 13-year-old hemophiliac boy was denied permission to attend the local school because he has AIDS. . . .''

Item: ''Federal scientists announced today that screening tests being used at blood banks around the country have been 'highly successful' in eliminating the AIDS 'virus' from the nation's blood supply. . . ."

Irrational fear, paranoia, and apocalyptic statements abound. The suggestion that casual contact can spread the disease (''He Chopped Green Beans & Roast Beef,'' read one sub-headline of a *New York Post* story about an AIDS victim who was a public school cook) contributed to both hysteria and homophobia. Rumors began to be induced by fear. Many newspapers and magazines started running cut-and-dry question-and-answer stories to cover and counter public fears. ABC's ''20/20'' showed Barbara Walters holding a toddler with AIDS in order to help show that the child posed no threat. Another problem with current news coverage is that the ''experts'' express different opinions.

In 1986, the *Washington Post* reported that 600,000 to 1.2 million persons might be infected, while the *Atlanta Constitution* put the number infected at 2 million, and reported that as many as one-third may get AIDS. In New York, where more than 2,000 people have already died from AIDS, careful reading of the *New York Times'* obituary page shows the use of euphemisms in place of the word ''AIDS,'' probably to lessen hysteria, and also to respect the feelings of the families.

In early November, 1985, the Soviet Union actually accused the C.I.A. of developing and spreading the AIDS ''virus'' during wide-range experiments in biological warfare. The major magazine *Literaturnaya Gazeta,* in an article headlined ''The Panic in the West,'' said that AIDS was spread from the U.S.

Since the first cases were identified in the U.S., AIDS has baffled the experts. There have been far more pervasive epidemics, certainly. Yet, one scientist, normally understated, has termed AIDS ''the disease of the century.''

"With AIDS," says Dr. Michael Gottlieb, a UCLA immunologist, "the word 'cure' is not yet in the vocabulary."

Gottlieb was among the first American physicians to notice something strange happening in the winter of 1981. In only three months, he treated four patients with an unusual lung infection called *Pneumocystis carinii PCP*, one of the "opportunistic" infections. He, as well as several other doctors working independently, recognized the outbreak of a previously unseen disease in record numbers. They all contacted the CDC in Atlanta, and the word was out.

There has been much controversy as to how far health officials can go in fighting disease. Many gay clubs, like the Mine Shaft in New York's Greenwich Village, a dark and raunchy bar where various sex acts were openly committed, had put public health officials on the spot as to how far they could go to stamp out AIDS. While the state clearly possesses the inherent power to protect the health and safety of their residents, at what point do such rules conflict with the adult's right to privacy? Are officials free to do anything to stamp out AIDS? Meanwhile such establishments in New York, San Francisco and other cities have been shut down.

In November, 1985, the New York State Public Health Council passed a 60-day emergency measure that would allow local officials to close "establishments" that "make facilities available" for "high risk" sex, meaning oral and anal sex. Health officials say this is no different from closing a disease-contaminated dairy. "The regulation is not directed at the individual engaged in the conduct, but at the commercial establishments and the activities that take place there," says State Health Department counsel Peter Millock.

For some, mere association with the specter of AIDS

can be lethal. In Houston, Patrick di Battista is a healthy, gay high school teacher who did community-relations work for a local AIDS foundation. When a magazine needed a photograph of an embracing gay couple that would run with an article about AIDS, di Battista agreed to pose. After the issue appeared, a local television personality presented a story criticizing the teacher's poor judgment in allowing his picture to be taken, even though his name was not used. The school district pulled di Battista out of his classroom and transferred him to a desk job.

The disease has developed more and more into a social issue. Los Angeles film and television actors, concerned with contracting the AIDS virus, have demanded the right to refuse to participate in scenes requiring heavy kissing, according to a Screen Actors' Guild policy statement. The performer, under the guild's new policy, has the right to refuse to film such scenes without penalty.

Despite what is now known about AIDS, the waves of fear many are now experiencing borders on hysteria. There are a number of reasons for this strong public reaction, and some are understandable and inevitable.

There are now many people at risk of developing the disease, although they may appear perfectly healthy now and may never get sick. No one knows how many that might be, but the U.S. Centers for Disease Control estimate 500,000 to one million, even quietly projecting an upper limit of two million. For the first time, there was talk of quarantining patients. *The Washington Post* reported that William Curran, professor of Legal Medicine at Harvard's Medical School, said that he was preparing standby regulations for cities to apply in confining AIDS patients who willfully persist in giving the disease to others. It would call first for a form of voluntary control, such as a signing of an agreement to inform partners that they have AIDS.

(After Rock Hudson died of AIDS on October 14, 1985, his 31-year-old lover, Mark Christian, sued Hudson's $3 million estate, claiming that he was exposed unknowingly to the disease. Christian claimed that everyone but he knew that Hudson had the disease.)

Dr. Curran stated, ''If a man keeps returning with gonorrhea, if he admits that he can't change his behavior, or if officials receive reports to that effect, then quarantine is in order.'' He advocated a scale of progressively more stringent confinement, from daily check-ins at an overnight hostel, to full-time custody in a guarded hospital. Said Curran, ''This is a plague and a menace, and I see nothing wrong with quarantine on a constitutional level.''

At least six bills were introduced in Congress regarding mandatory blood testing; all require the results to be reported to the proper health agencies. Another bill makes the willful spreading of AIDS a felony. Some government officials stated that hotel rooms in high-risk areas should be inspected regularly, with room warrants.

Many insurance companies, employers and social-service agencies are shunning healthy homosexuals, making AIDS a social-political disease instead of merely a medical one. Fear of an epidemic and panic prevail.

AIDS WITHIN PRISON WALLS

There is a growing fear of the spread of AIDS in prisons. The concern gravitates especially around the inmate population who participate in homosexual activities and use intravenous drugs. Trapped inside four walls and closely quartered with other convicts, prisoners are scared.

Guards are also frightened—specifically, that if a prisoner with AIDS bites or cuts them, they might contract AIDS.

The cases of AIDS in prisons jumped 61 percent in

1986. Prisoners dying from AIDS has created the phrase, ''A new death row.'' Most cases are in New York, New Jersey, and Florida.

Condoms are being distributed for the men's sexual activity, and intravenous drugs are ferreted out, to cut down the incidence of AIDS.

When prisoners do contract this dread disease, they are quickly released into the public mainstream, or into city hospitals. Prison officials state they have no facilities to cope with sick and dying prisoners with AIDS, and that prisons contain all the ingredients for disaster. The public is worried.

Dr. Samuel Broder, chief of Clinical Oncology at the National Cancer Institute near Washington, D.C., is optimistic that the NCI and private pharmaceutical companies can develop new compounds for AIDS. Of course, chemical medicine is very profitable, both for doctors and pharmaceutical companies.

''It's a (potential) billion-dollar market,'' says Dominic Liuzzi, an ICN Pharmaceuticals Vice-President.

The U.S. Food and Drug Administration is testing many drugs experimentally. Two drugs, namely, isoprinosine and ribaviron, reportedly were selling on the black market for as much as ten times their retail value.

As with any such drugs, there are potentially dangerous side effects—anemia, liver damage, etc.

John Lounsbury, a Person With AIDS, gives this depressing comment, ''The worst thing that can happen by taking the drug is that you lose your life. Without it, you die anyway.'' This is the prevailing belief.

The results of testing are being closely watched, not only by Persons With AIDS, but also by ICN Pharmaceuticals, Inc. and Newport Pharmaceuticals, Inc.—the Orange County (CA) manufacturers of ribaviron and isoprinosine, respectively.

''These people are dying, and they're being offered absolutely no hope,'' said Steven Webb, assistant to a New York physician who has traveled to Tijuana, Mexico, and purchased the two drugs for patients. ''It's a life-and-death situation,'' he said.

Disease-free Americans have been going to Mexico for these drugs out of fear that they may develop the disease. U.S. Customs officials in San Diego announced in October, 1985, that they would permit Americans to bring back from Tijuana limited amounts of isoprinosine and ribaviron —so long as the drugs are for personal use. This was a significant policy shift by the F.D.A. and the U.S. Customs. These drugs are also available in Europe, but it is the Mexican border cities where most U.S. citizens go. A number of knowledgeable physicians have cautioned against the use of these two drugs. Some fear that isoprinosine might actually do more harm than good, because the drug stimulates the growth of new healthy cells, which actually accelerates the progress of AIDS—because the AIDS virus feeds off the healthy cells.

The federal government is now looking for two types of drugs. One drug should kill the virus without killing the patient. The other should repair the patient's immune system. The problem is that not enough is known about how the T-cells react to the AIDS virus.

A spokesman for the Centers for Disease Control said, ''When we develop the new vaccine, every man, woman and child in the U.S. should take it, to keep from getting AIDS.''

However, Surgeon General C. Everett Koop announced in March, 1987, that it is unlikely that we will see a vaccine cure before the year 2000.

In October, 1986, the press announced ''A Ray of Hope in the Fight Against AIDS'' with an experimental drug called azidothymidine (AZT). No cure was promised, and there are dangerous side effects. The drug manufacturer —Burroughs Wellcome Company—admits to the public, on their AIDS drug hotline, that the side effects include severe anemia (loss of red blood cells; transfusions may be needed); headaches; nausea; mild confusion and anxiety; skin rashes and itching; lower white blood cell count, and the suppression of bone-marrow production. The company admits it has no idea of the long-term side effects, and says, "It can be used only when there is *Pneumocystic carinii* pneumonia."

On March 20, 1987, the F.D.A. approved the sale of this drug—sold under the brand name of Retrovir. Although AZT is *not* a cure for AIDS, in clinical studies it has prolonged the lives of victims of *Pneumocystis carinii* pneumonia, a rare infection associated with AIDS. The drug is very expensive, with a year's supply costing between $7,000 and $10,000, at this time.

In May, 1986, a California report stated that the average life expectancy of AIDS patients may range from eighteen months to as little as two months, depending on which of its many forms the lethal disease takes.

The devastating lung disease called *Pneumocystis carinii* pneumonia accounts for more AIDS deaths than any other infection, and it strikes nearly 60 per cent of all AIDS patients. About 35 percent are stricken with the skin cancer called Kaposi's sarcoma, and 6 percent have both. Toxoplasmosis is caused by a protozoan organism called *Toxoplasma gondii*, and is a very deadly AIDS infection.

The cost of caring for AIDS patients is becoming monumental—at least $100 million was spent in 1986 in California alone. In Los Angeles, the average hospital stay is eighteen days and the cost reaches $109,000 before death.

On February 4, 1987, the star Liberace died in Palm Springs, California. No doctor was in attendance, and the cause of death was given as a combination of heart disease, anemia and emphysema. However, after an autopsy, the coroner's report gave the cause of death as ''Infection triggered by AIDS.''

Conflicts at the Centers for Disease Control made the news in 1987. Reporter Jonathan Kwitny of *The Wall Street Journal* found that ''ego clashes, professional jealousies, and perhaps worse'' have crippled the C.D.C.'s AIDS laboratories, which have been the subject of allegations of ''hampered research, political meddling, and even sabotaged experiments.'' What would the motivations be for such acts? One scientist stated, ''AIDS research has attracted a certain type of personality. There's a lot of power to be had. The C.D.C. controls a lot of money. There are a lot of egos involved and they are clashing.''

It was stated in various publications that in South Africa, Persons With AIDS must leave the country. England is refusing to admit known Persons With AIDS. These regulations may create problems, because in many cases AIDS is difficult to diagnose. Needed are not only visible symptoms but laboratory results.

California biologist Bruce Voeller found that certain spermicides are capable of killing sexually transmitted organisms. Reportedly, he proposed to Dr. Curran, head of the C.D.C., that a study be done of these spermicides on the AIDS virus, but Dr. Curran refused. Voeller later conducted the study with the help of a technician at the C.D.C., which showed that the spermicide killed the AIDS virus in vitro. But no public announcement was ever made, because the spermicide is something you can get in the drugstore. The spermicide is benzalkonium chloride.

The special virus which it is believed causes AIDS was called HTLV-III, until recently. *Time* magazine reported that the new and preferred term for the AIDS-causing agent is HIV, or human immunodeficiency virus. This suggests that a whole group of immune-deficiency related illnesses will be lumped into one broad category, to which the label of AIDS can be given. The broad spectrum proposed by the C.D.C. (''Mononucleosislike symptom'') —means that any viral immune-deficiency disease can come under the name of AIDS. This would increase the AIDS fatality figures considerably, add to the epidemic scare, and create the demand for huge sums for research and cure.

Reagan Finally Speaks on AIDS. On the *NBC Nightly News* with Tom Brokaw, broadcast on April 1, 1987, White House correspondent Andrea Mitchell reported, ''Officials confirm that the President has never talked to the Surgeon General about AIDS or read the report that Dr. Koop sent him last October.'' On April 3, a White House press officer confirmed through *Frontier* magazine that Mitchell's statement was correct. The Reagan administration has finally addressed AIDS because it has become a major health issue.

Surgeon General C. Everett Koop said that he does not have sufficient money to convene a national meeting needed to deal with the rising cost of dealing with AIDS. Without such a meeting, Koop said, ''The cost in both dollars and personnel will simply overwhelm our hospital system and have enormous potential for bankrupting a community's health system.''

In speaking before the College of Physicians in March, 1987, President Reagan addressed the issue of AIDS, by commenting on the pressure to inform youth on the facts about AIDS, and to make condoms more readily available. His comment emphasized teaching moral values, and abstinence, rather than mere prevention through this mechanical device.

In 1978–79, an experimental vaccine, aimed at the prevention of Hepatitis-B, was administered in New York City and San Francisco to gay men. The vaccine was obtained from individuals who had hepatitis. At that time, there was little testing for the purity of blood, thus no way to recognize contamination, because the AIDS virus was unknown. The question arises, Is it possible that the blood of these donors was contaminated?

On the ABC network program called *Ask Dr. Ruth*, one week was devoted to education on AIDS. On February 4–5, 1987, the guest was Matilde Krim, M.D., who had done pioneering work with AIDS. She stated that a Hepatitis-B vaccine was tested in 1978–79 in the gay communities in New York and San Francisco; the vaccine was given without charge in this federal experiment; and the serum was derived from the blood of Africans who had hepatitis. Her theory was that was how AIDS found its way into the gay community.

Dr. J. Anthony Morris also comments on this issue. He is a leading virologist for 35 years who has worked with the National Institutes of Health, Walter Reed Hospital, and the Food and Drug Administration in connection with its research on vaccine. He has a theory that he is careful to preface as "speculative."

"The AIDS virus began to appear in homosexuals around 1979. That was immediately following tests of the first hepatitis vaccine." That vaccine was tested on homosexual populations. Soon after the completion of those tests, AIDS was first detected. Dr. Morris points out that today "the commercially marketed vaccine is manufactured in the same manner." As the technique for identifying the AIDS virus was developed only recently, "there is no way of telling how many people received hepatitis vaccines that may have been infected with the AIDS virus," writes Gary Null in an article in *Penthouse* magazine (Part XII, "Medical Genocide").

Dr. Morris also states that the unquestioned pursuit of an AIDS vaccine is an alarming trend, and may be self-serving on the part of some of the scientists and governmental agencies involved. "They are asking for a couple billion dollars a year. This is nonsense. You don't need two billion dollars to do this work."

Terry Krieger, a Washington journalist who has been researching AIDS, explained in *The Miami Herald* that "a syndrome is a set of symptoms that reflect a disease. For example, fever, nasal congestion, muscle pain, and stomach upset may reflect influenza. In AIDS, however, the symptoms themselves represent over a dozen diseases, none of which is new. Moreover, not all AIDS patients have the same diseases, and the death rates for AIDS patients depend on which diseases they have. So, AIDS is not a single syndrome, but several conditions resulting from severe damage to the body's immune system, which defends the body from the disease." Furthermore, not only are the statistics concerning AIDS inflated, there is also evidence that the rate of increase of AIDS is on the decline, says Null.

Project Inform, a San Francisco-based concern, is giving out information as to where *individuals* can purchase drugs to treat AIDS that they cannot otherwise obtain in this country from their doctors. The 15-page paper (dated November, 1986), they mail out is entitled "Federally

Unapproved Medications for Treatment of AIDS and Aids-Related Conditions (ARC); How to Get Them; How to Bring Them Home; How to Use Them."

Details on how to smuggle across the Mexican border more capsules than are allowed, and details on dosages, etc., are included in the papers. Some AIDS patients are so desperate they will do anything—even follow these instructions of how to get illegal quantities of these questionable drugs from over the border.

The doctor of the future
will give no medicine
but will interest his patients
in the care of the human frame,
in diet, and in the cause and
prevention of disease.

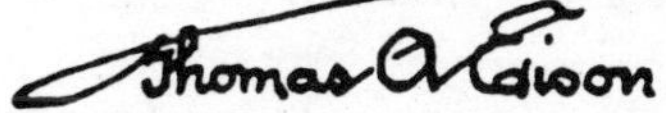

Thomas A. Edison

Laughter—along with hope,
faith, love, will to live, creativity—
can be regarded as an important
resource in any strategy of recovery or,
indeed, in prompting good health.

Norman Cousins

RECOMMENDED READING

General Health:

Airola, Paavo, Ph.D. *Meat for B-12?* Nutrition Health Review, (Summer 1983): 13.

Allen, Hannah. *The Happy Truth About Protein*. Austin, TX: Life Science, 1976.

————. "Lesson No. 33, Why We Should Not Eat Animal Products in Any Form." In *The Life Science Health System*, by T. C. Fry. Austin, TX: Life Science, 1984.

Ames, Bruce N. "Dietary Carcinogens and Anti-Carcinogens." *Science*, 23 September 1983: 1256.

Bach, Edward. *Heal Thyself*. London: Daniel, 1946.

Barnett, Iris. *Candida: How I Overcame It Naturally, Without Drugs*. 1985.

Bealle, Morris A. *The Drug Story*. Spanish Fork, UT: The Hornet's Nest, 1949.

————. *The New Drug Story*. Washington, D.C.: Columbia Publishing Co., 1958.

Beiler, Henry G., M.D. *Food Is Your Best Medicine*. New York: Random House, 1965.

Benowicz, Robert. *Vitamins and You*. New York: Berkley Books, 1983.

Benton, Mike. "Lesson No. 30, Sugars and Other Sweeteners May Be Worse Than Bad." In *The Life Science Health System*, by T. C. Fry. Austin, TX: Life Science, 1984.

Bragg, Paul. *The Shocking Truth About Water*. Santa Barbara, CA: Health Science, 1985.

Bricklin, Mark. *Rodale's Encyclopedia of Natural Home Remedies*. Emmaus, PA: Rodale Press, 1982.

Cantwell, Alan, Jr., M.D. *A.I.D.S., The Mystery and the Solution*. Los Angeles: Aries Rising Press, 1983.

Cousins, Norman. *Anatomy of an Illness*. New York: Bantam Books, 1979.

Crook, William G., M.D. *The Yeast Connection*. Jackson, TN: Professional Books, 1985.

Heritage, Ford. *Composition and Facts About Foods*. Mokelumne Hill, CA: Health Research, 1968.

Inglis, Bruce. *Natural Medicine*. Glasgow, Great Britain: William Collins & Sons, 1979.

Jensen, Bernard, D.C. *Tissue Cleansing Through Bowel Management*. Escondido, CA: Bernard Jensen, 6th edition, 1981.

Kime, Zane R., M.D. *Sunlight Could Save Your Life*. Penryn, CA: World Health, 1980.

Kushi, Michio. *The Book of Macrobiotics*. Tokyo, Japan: Japan Publications, 1977.

————. *Oriental Diagnosis*. London, England: Red Moon, 1978.

Leonardo, Bianca, Ph.D. *Cancer and Other Diseases Caused by Meat Consumption—Here's the Evidence*. Santa Monica, CA: Leaves of Healing Publications, 1979.

Longwood, William. *Poisons in Your Food*. New York: Pyramid, 1969.

Malstrom, Stan D. *Own Your Own Body*. New Canaan, CT: Pivot Health, 1980.

Mindell, Earl, Ph.D. *Earl Mindell's Pill Bible*. New York: Bantam, 1984.

————. *The Missing Vitamin—B-15*. New York: Fred Jordan Books, 1979.

Muramoto, Naboru. *Healing Ourselves*. New York: Avon Books, 1973.

Parham, Barbara. *What's Wrong with Eating Meat?* Denver, CO: Ananda Marga Publications, 1979.

Pauling, Linus. *How to Live Longer and Feel Better.* New York: W. H. Freeman & Co., 1986.

Rose, Elizabeth. *Lady of Gray Healing Candida*. Santa Monica: Butterfly Publishers, 1985.

Shelton, Herbert, Ph.D. *Food Combining Made Easy.* San Antonio, TX: Dr. Shelton's Health School, 1951.

Singer, Peter, and Mason, Jim. *Animal Factories.* Bridgeport, CT: Natural Hygiene Press, 1980.

Teague, Terri K., and Jackson, Mildred. *The Handbook of Alternatives to Chemical Medicine*. Oakland, CA, 1984.

Tilden, John H., M.D. *Toxemia Explained*. Denver: Health Research, 1926.

Verett, Jacqueline, and Carper, Jean. *Eating May be Hazardous to Your Health*. New York: Simon & Schuster, 1974.

Waerland, Are. *Health Is Your Birthright*. Bern, Switzerland: Humanata Publishers, circa 1945.

Waerland, Ebba. *Cancer, a Disease of Civilization*. Ontario, Canada: Provoker Press, 1980.

Walker, Norman, W., D.Sc., M.D. *Colon Health*. Phoenix, AZ: O'Sullivan Woodside & Co., 1979.

Weiner, Michael A., Ph.D. *Maximum Immunity*. Boston: Houghton Mifflin Co., 1986.

Welsh, Philip J., D.D.S., N.D., and Leonardo, Bianca, Ph.D. *Freedom from Arthritis Through Nutrition*. Santa Monica, CA: Arthritis Research, 1980.

Health Cookbooks:

————. *The Ananda Cookbook*. Nevada City, CA: Ananda Publishers, 1985.

Bagg, Elmer. *Cooking Without a Grain of Salt*. New York: Bantam Books, 1964.

Bragg, Paul and Patricia. *Gourmet Health Recipes for Life Extension*. Santa Barbara, CA: Health Science, 1984.

Connolly, Pat. *The Candida Albicans Yeast-Free Cookbook*. New Canaan, CT: Keats Publishing, Inc., 1985.

Diamond, Harvey and Marilyn. *Fit for Life*. New York: Warner Books, 1985.

Gregory, Patricia. *Bean Banquets from Boston to Bombay*. Santa Barbara, CA: Woodbridge Press, 1984.

Hurd, Frank J., D.C., and Rosalie, B.S. *Ten Talents*. Chisholm, MN: Dr. and Mrs. Frank J. Hurd, 1984.

Kloss, Jethro. *Back to Eden Cookbook, The*. Loma Linda, CA: Back to Eden Publications, 1981.

Kushi, Esko, and Kushi, Aveline. *The Changing Seasons: Macrobiotic Cookbook*. Boston: Avery, 1985.

Rockwell, Sally. *Coping with Candida Cookbook*. Seattle, WA: 1984.

———. *Vegetarian Cookbook*. Melon Park, CA: Sunset International, Lane Publishing, 1983.

Walker, Norman W., M.D. *Fresh Vegetable and Fruit Juices*. Phoenix, AZ: O'Sullivan Woodside & Co., 1981.

Herbal Books:

———. *A Barefoot Doctor's Manual*. Philadelphia, PA: Running Press, 1977.

Grieve, M. *A Modern Herbal*. New York: Donner Publications (two volumes), 1971.

Kloss, Jethro. *Back to Eden*. Loma Linda, CA: Back to Eden Publications, 1984.

Rose, Jeanne. *Rose's Herbal Guide to Inner Health*. New York: Grosset & Dunlap, 1979.

Royal, Penny L. *Herbally Yours*. Payson, UT: Sound Nutrition, 1982.

Mental/Spiritual Books:

Eddy, Mary Baker. *Science and Health with Key to the Scriptures* & other works. Boston, MA: Christian Science Publishing Society.

Gawain, Shakti. *Creative Visualization*. New York: Bantam New Age Books.

Harrison, John. *Love Your Disease—It's Keeping You Healthy*. Angus and Robertson Publishers, London.

Hay, Louise L. *You Can Heal Your Life*; Cassette Tape: *Self-Healing* and other works. Santa Monica, CA: Hay House.

(There are innumerable other books in the field of spiritual healing.)

Books offered/published by Tree of Life
P.O. Box 126, Joshua Tree, CA 92252-0126

Cancer and Other Diseases Caused by Meat Consumption —Here's the Evidence.

Deep Thoughts on War and Peace & Other Essays on the Vegetarian Way of Life.

*The Benjamin Franklin Success and Happiness Perpetual Date
   Book.*
Natural Nutrition: Answer to Cancer.
A Treasury of Health Wisdom.
The Unknown Life of Jesus Christ by Nicholas Notovitch.

VEGETARIAN SOCIETY, INC., P.O. Box 126, Joshua Tree,
   CA 92252-0126. For more information on the vegetarian diet
   and way of life, please send a SASE.

APPENDIX

Most diets indicate the need for potential nutrient supplementation. DAILY NUTRIENT INTAKE, WITHOUT SUPPLEMENTS, is *BELOW* the RDA (Recommended Daily Allowance) FOR:

1. VITAMIN A

a. Low intake encourages night blindness, poor wound healing, dry skin and hair, impaired immunity to infection, poor mucopolysaccharide synthesis.

b. Constituent of rhodopsin (visual pigment); maintenance of epithelial tissues, role in mucopolysaccharide synthesis (tissue cement).

2. VITAMIN B_1 (Thiamine)

a. Low intake increases risk to glucose intolerance, changes in behavior (hyperactivity, irritability, mood swings), beriberi (peripheral nerve changes, edema, heart failure), fatigue and low exercise potential.

3. VITAMIN B_2 (Riboflavin)

a. Low intake reddens lips, cracks at corner of mouth (chellosis), lesions of the eye, poor utilization of fat.

4. VITAMIN B_3 (Niacin)

a. Low intake: Pellagra (skin and gastrointestinal lesions, nervous mental disorders), impaired neuro-hormone synthesis, poor circulation.

5. VITAMIN B_6 (Pyridoxine)

a. Low intake encourages musculo-skeletal problems such as carpel tunnel syndrome, arteriosclerosis in susceptible males and all contraceptive-induced depression, as well as poor dream recall, muscular twitching, kidney stones.

b. Essential for not only the proper metabolism of protein but also as a coenzyme in brain chemistry for proper normalization of neurotransmitters.

6. VITAMIN B_{12} (Cyanocobalamin)

a. Low intake can lead to blood and metabolic problems, particularly in lactating mothers or diabetics; pernicious anemia, neurological disorders, problems in fat metabolism and red blood cell synthesis.

b. Vegetarians may not be getting adequate Vitamin B_{12}.

7. FOLIC ACID

a. Low intake can lead to neurological problems, especially in pregnant women, elevated uric acid levels, anemia, gastrointestinal disturbances, red tongue, diarrhea, mood, mind and memory changes in the elderly.

8. PANTOTHENIC ACID

a. Low intake: Fatigue, poor resistance to infection, adrenal exhaustion, sleep disturbances, impaired coordination, nausea, allergies, lowered tolerance to stress, inflammation—general or local.

9. BIOTIN

a. Low intake: Fatigue, nausea, depression, dermatitis, poor hair growth, muscular pains.

10. CHOLINE

a. Low intake can induce fatty liver, a decrease in brain acetylcholine, which results in memory loss and symptoms such as tardive dyskinesia, as well as reduced HDL (High-Density Lipoprotein) levels in the blood.

b. The best source is egg or soy lecithin—at least 13% phosphotydl choline content.

11. INOSITOL

a. Low intake: Arteriosclerosis, high level cholesterol, stroke, constipation, dizziness, glaucoma, baldness, liver problems, asthma gastritis, overweight and obesity.

12. VITAMIN C
(Ascorbic Acid)

a. Low intake increases risk to cardiovascular, gastrointestinal, endocrine and periodontal imbalance.

b. Can reduce blood cholesterol levels and increase bile production.

c. Can strengthen the key lymphocyte system increasing the body's defense against viral and other infections.

13. VITAMIN E

a. Low intake can encourage free radical pathology and accelerated destruction of cell membranes associated with the aging process. This process may result in arteriosclerosis, cancer or skin wrinkling.

b. Affects the cardiovascular, respiratory, endocrine systems, and bone formation.

14. VITAMIN D

a. Low intake can encourage bone deformities in children and osteomalacia in adults.

b. People who consume fortified milk and dairy products and processed foods take in an average of 3,300 units of D daily. Extra supplementation with D is unnecessary.

Sunshine is the best source of Vitamin D.

15. LOW INTAKE OF VITAMINS AND MINERALS

reduces the metabolic competency and increases the risk of many degenerative diseases. The first symptoms include gastrointestinal problems, sleep disturbances, change in energy level, and personality changes, which may be aggressive in nature.

FOODS HIGH IN ESSENTIAL NUTRIENTS

Foods are listed in approximate amounts supplied by average servings, highest first and decreasing as one reads down. The authors have omitted meats and milk, as they are not recommended. Eggs should be fertile. Cottage cheese is found in several groups; it is better to make your own; the commercial variety usually has salt and other harmful ingredients. We include a recipe for making your own cottage cheese from raw milk.

PROTEIN

Essential Fatty Acids
Soybeans (dry)
Fish
Vegetable patty
Cottage cheese

AMINO ACIDS

Iso-leucine
Fish
Soybeans
Soy protein
Vegetable patty
Eggs
Cottage cheese
Baked beans

Lysine
Fish
Soy protein
Soybeans
Cottage cheese
Baked beans
Eggs
Vegetable patty
Oatmeal

Methionine/cystine
Fish
Eggs
Cottage cheese
Soybeans
Soy protein
Vegetable patty
Sardines
Yogurt

Phenylalanine/tyrosine
Soy protein
Soybeans
Fish
Vegetable patty
Eggs
Cottage cheese
Baked beans
Almonds (not roasted,
    not salted or sugared)

Threonine
Fish
Soy protein
Soybeans
Cottage cheese
Baked beans
Vegetable patty

Tryptophan
Soy protein
Soybeans
Fish
Eggs
Vegetable patty
Cottage cheese
Mixed nuts (not roasted,
    not salted)
Baked beans

Valine
Fish
Soy protein
Soybeans
Eggs

Vegetable patty
Cottage cheese
Baked beans

VITAMINS

Vitamin A
Dark green, leafy vegetables
Cantaloupe
Sweet potato
Carrots
Spinach, chard
Tomato
Eggs

Vitamin B_1
Soybeans (dry)
Sunflower seeds (not roasted
    or salted)
Fortified cereals
Brazil nuts (not roasted
    or salted)
Oatmeal

Vitamin B_2
Mushrooms
Fortified cereals
Eggs
Cottage cheese
Spinach

Niacin
Salmon, tuna (fresh preferred)
Halibut (fresh preferred)
All bran
Mushrooms
Other fish

Vitamin B_6
Soybeans
Fresh salmon (salt free)
Molasses
Wheat bran
Cod
Sunflower seeds

Vitamin B_{12}
Oysters
Salmon
Fresh sole filet

Pantothenic Acid
Eggs
Soybeans
Broccoli
Mushrooms
Haddock

Folacin (folic acid)
Asparagus
Lettuce
Spinach
Orange juice
Legumes (peas, beans, lentils)

Vitamin C
Guava
Broccoli
Green peppers
Brussels sprouts
Cantaloupe
Dark green leafy vegetables
Citrus fruit or juice
Strawberries, fresh
Cabbage
Watermelon

Vitamin E
Soybean oil
Corn or cottonseed oil
Wheat germ
Margarine
Mayonnaise
Salmon steak, broiled

MINERALS

Calcium
Broccoli
Dark green leafy vegetables

Cheese
Molasses
Legumes
Almonds
Cottage cheese
Brazil nuts

Chromium
Corn

Copper
Eggs
Molasses

Iodine
Ocean Fish
Shellfish
Spinach

Iron
Prune juice
Soybeans
Baked beans
Spinach
Eggs

Magnesium
Soybeans
Wheat germ
Cashews
Almonds
Brazil nuts
Baked beans
Molasses
Dark green leafy
  vegetables

Manganese
Wheat germ

Phosphorus
Tuna
Wheat germ
Soybeans
Brazil nuts

Potassium
Soybeans
Cantaloupe
Tomatoes
Sweet potato
Avocado
Raisins
Banana
Halibut, sole
Baked beans
Molasses
Mushrooms
White potatoes

Selenium
Wheat germ
Legumes
Eggs
Onions
Garlic

Zinc
Oatmeal
Fish
Dried beans
Bran
Tuna

ANALYSIS OF POLLEN CONTENT

VITAMINS
1. Provitamin A
2. B_1 Thiamine
3. B_2 Riboflavin
4. Niacin
5. B_6 Group
6. Pantothenic acid
7. Biotin
8. B_{12} (cyanocobalamin)

9. Folic acid
10. Choline
11. Inositol
12. Vitamin C
13. Vitamin D
14. Vitamin E
15. Vitamin K
16. Rutin

MINERALS
1. Calcium
2. Phosphorus
3. Potassium
4. Sulphur
5. Sodium
6. Chlorine
7. Magnesium
8. Iron
9. Manganese
10. Copper
11. Iodine
12. Zinc
13. Silicon
14. Molybdenum
15. Boron
16. Titanium

ENZYMES, CO-ENZYMES
1. Amylase
2. Diastase
3. Saccharase
4. Pectase
5. Phosphatase
6. Catalase
7. Disphorase
8. Cozymase
9. Cytochrome systems
10. Lactic dehydrogenase
11. Succinic dehydrogenase
12. 24 oxidoreductases
13. 21 transferases
14. 33 hydrolases
15. 11 lyases
16. 5 isomerases
17. Pepsin
18. Trypsin

PROTEIN/AMINO ACIDS
1. Isoleucine
2. Leucine
3. Lysine
4. Methionine
5. Phenylalanine
6. Threonine
7. Typtophan
8. Valine
9. Histidine
10. Arginine
11. Cystine
12. Tyrosine
13. Alanine
14. Aspartic acid
15. Glutamic acid
16. Hydroxyproline
17. Proline
18. Serine

OTHERS
1. Nucleic acids
2. Flavonoids
3. Phenolic acids
4. Tarpenes
5. Nucleosides
6. Auxins
7. Fructose
8. Glucose
9. Brassins
10. Gibberellins
11. Kinins
12. Vernine
13. Guanine
14. Xanthine
15. Hypoxalthine
16. Nuclein
17. Amines
18. Lecithin
19. Zanthophylls
20. Crocetin
21. Zeaxanthin
22. Mycopene
23. Hexodecanal
24. Alpha-amino-butyric-acid

25. Monoglycerides
26. Diglycerides
27. Triglycerides
28. Pentosans

PROTEIN
Excess protein leads to:
1. Increased risk of kidney problems
2. Increased risk of liver problems
3. Elevated blood cholesterol
4. Bone calcium loss leading to osteoporosis and periodontal disease
5. Possible symptoms associated with excess protein intake are:
   a. Water retention, general puffiness, swollen ankles
   b. Menstrual difficulties — painful, overflow, etc.
   c. Constipation
   d. Belching and bloating during and directly after meals
   e. Restlessness
   f. Fatigue after eating
   g. Allergies and food sensitivities
   h. Poor endurance, general sluggishness
   i. Bladder and yeast infections
   j. Painful joints
   k. Lower back pains
   l. Arthritis

**Deficient protein
leads to:**
1. Lower immune defense to infection
2. Wasting of muscle mass
3. Poor wound healing
4. Lowered metabolic rate
5. Infertility
6. Increased susceptibility to degenerative disease
7. Accelerated aging

8. Mind, mood and memory problems; forgetfulness, depression, poor comprehension, etc.
9. Extreme fatigue
10. Anemia
11. Inadequate balance of essential amino acids inhibits the utilization of protein in the body

Requirements:
1. Most people need between 60-80 grams of good quality protein daily: Fish, poultry (no skin), eggs (poached, soft-boiled), dairy (low-fat milk, cultured milk products, low-fat cheeses), lean meat, legume and grain combinations (rice, corn, beans, soy, millet, lentils, limas, wheat berries, rye, etc.). Vegetarians will delete the meat, fish, poultry.

CARBOHYDRATES
(Unrefined sugars, fiber)
1. Bran-based fiber from corn, wheat, rice or oats is desired to increase intestinal transit time of food.
2. Detoxification program may be required when beginning a higher fiber diet.
3. START SLOWLY and gradually build up unrefined carbohydrate enrichment (whole grains, legumes, beans, fresh vegetables, whole fruits).

**Excessive dietary
sugars:**
1. Increases risk of appendicitis, colon cancer, diverticulosis, hemorrhoids, constipation, allergies, reabsorption of toxic waste products into circulation

which encourages the development of degenerative diseases such as heart disease and arthritis.
2. Increases risk of adult-onset diabetes, mood and behavior changes, hypoglycemia and dysglycemia, obesity and its related problems.
3. Total dietary sugars from natural sources and from sucrose-laden foods, including hidden sugars found in processed foods, must be controlled.
4. Remember that hidden sugar in processed foods is a major contributor to total daily sugar intake.
5. Possible symptoms associated with high dietary sugar intake are:
   a. Nervousness
   b. Irritability
   c. Exhaustion
   d. Faintness and dizziness
   e. Tremors and cold sweats
   f. Depression
   g. Headaches
   h. Digestive disturbances
   i. Insomnia; inability to fall asleep once awake
   j. Cravings for sugar and/or alcohol
   k. Mood swings
   l. Constant worrying
   m. Unprovoked anxieties
   n. Mental confusion
   o. Internal trembling
   p. Rapid pulse
   q. Frequent sighing and yawning

FAT
Excessive fat (total) consumption
1. Increases risk to heart disease, certain cancers, obesity, sugar

intolerance, food sensitivities and allergies, gastrointestinal problems, liver and endocrine imbalance.
2. Possible symptoms associated with high fat intake:
   a. Light colored stool (gray, white, yellow)
   b. Chronic constipation
   c. Dry or oily skin; acne or eczema
   d. Digestive disturbances (gas, bloating, belching, sour taste, food repeats)
   e. Bad breath and body odor, feet smell
   f. Tiredness after eating
   g. Extreme fatigue
   h. General puffiness; swollen ankles
   i. Male and female reproductive problems (menstrual irregularity and pain; prostate pain, infertility)
   j. Weight problems (cannot gain or lose weight)
   k. Dryness of hair
   l. High cholesterol
   m. Gallstones
   n. Poor circulation
   o. Menopausal problems (hot flashes, etc.)
   p. Intolerance to sugar and fats (mood swings, cry easily, tense, irritable)
   q. Changes in mood, mind and memory (poor retention), inability to concentrate, blurred vision.
   r. Bloated feeling two to three hours after eating.
3. Fat should comprise no more than 25% of your total caloric intake
4. Saturated animal fat appears to have a more important effect

upon raising blood cholesterol levels and causing platelet adhesions which increases risk of clots (thrombosis)

5. Hydrogenated fats (margarines, shortenings, refined vegetable oils) also contribute to increased risk of heart disease, elevated cholesterol, obesity, liver problems and some cancers. These heated oils are poorly assimilated and can block bile production. Bile is one of the major ways the body rids itself of cholesterol.

6. Alfalfa seedmeal and guar gum have a cholesterol-lowering effect on the blood. Norwegian cod liver oil (cold water fish only) has a blood-thinning effect where platelet adhesion is marked.

Low essential fat intake such as linoleic and arachidonic acids

1. Reduce necessary hormone and prostaglandin synthesis
2. Encourage skin problems
3. Encourage reproductive problems
4. Encourage platelet adhesion
5. Encourage central nervous system weakness
6. Very low dietary fat intake over long periods of time, as well as very high saturated fat diets which may block the appropriate uptake and utilization of the essential fats, can produce the above effects (1-5)
7. Possible symptoms associated with low essential fatty acid intake are:
   a. Enlarged and inflamed prostate
   b. Menopausal problems (hot flashes)
   c. Suppressed menstruation
   d. Dry skin and hair
   e. Nerve degeneration
   f. Poor endurance; low tolerance for exercise
   g. Eczema and psoriasis
   h. Depressed immunity to infectious
   i. Poor wound healing due to poor utilization of zinc
8. Sources of essential fatty acids are cold pressed vegetable oils, Norwegian cod liver oil, Evening Primrose Oil, whole grains, small amounts of unroasted nuts and seeds, limited amounts of unrefined seed and fruit oils, avocados,

SALT
Excessive intake

1. Increases potential of blood pressure problems
2. Increases risk of arteriosclerosis, kidney failure and stroke
3. Do not salt food before tasting since this increases salt intake considerably
4. Processed foods have a very high salt content, which contributes to hidden salt consumption in the diet

Unsupplemented ratios sodium to potassium ratio affects:

1. Fluid balance
2. Cardiovascular function
3. Reproduction
4. Urological system (kidney and bladder)
5. Hormone balance (adrenal glands)

6. Possible symptoms associated with altered dietary sodium to potassium ratio are:
   a. Chronic fatigue, feeling drowsy
   b. Bruising easily
   c. Cold hands and feet; must use extra clothing
   d. Shortness of breath with slightest exertion
   e. Requires extra sleep
   f. Lowered endurance; low exercise potential
   g. General puffiness: swollen ankles
   h. Spills protein in urine
   i. Known allergies, asthma and chronic sniffles
   j. Easy weight gain (several pounds overnight)
   k. Increased morning stiffness, painful joints
   l. Heart palpitations
   m. Chest pain, leg fatigue
   n. Persistent high blood pressure (high sodium)
   o. Low blood pressure
   p. Difficulty urinating, burning, great frequency
   q. Menopausal symptoms (hot flashes, etc.)
   r. Before menstrual periods feel nervous, depressed
   s. Eyes are sensitive to bright lights

Calcium to phosphorus ratio affects:

1. Bone formation
2. Cardiovascular function (heart, veins, arteries)
3. Musculo-skeletal system
4. Endocrine system
5. Possible symptoms associated with low dietary Calcium to Phosphorus ratio are:
   a. Bone loss—osteoporosis, periodontal disease, osteo-arthritis
   b. kidneys, stiffness in joints and muscles, mood, mind and memory problems due to poor circulation or hypo-parathyroidism, depressed immunity to infections due to poor utilization of zinc, prostate problems
6. High phosphorus, low calcium diets are due to use of excessive meats, fabricated foods and soft drinks (sugared or synthetically sweetened)
7. Increased complex carbohydrates, low fat and cultured dairy products as opposed to hard cheese and whole milk create a more favorable balance of calcium to phosphorus in diet

Calcium to magnesium ratio affects:

1. Smooth muscle integrity
2. Cardiovascular system, gastro-intestinal function, muscular/skeletal system
3. Possible associated symptoms with high Calcium to Magnesium ratio are:
   a. Coronary artery collapse (vasospasm)
   b. Muscle cramping
   c. Poor bowel regularity (constipation)
   d. Elevated triglycerides
   e. Missed heartbeats
   f. Kidney stones
   g. Muscle stiffness
   h. Menstrual problems (cramps, depression)